Christy M. Ponticelli
Editor

Gateways to Improving Lesbian Health and Health Care: Opening Doors

Pre-publication
REVIEWS,
COMMENTARIES,
EVALUATIONS . . .

This volume contains information that could prove vital to your health or the health of a loved one. This book is especially important for health providers to read so that they can do their jobs more effectively. It presents a wide array of cases and data about lesbians and their health from throughout the United States and Canada–rural and urban, multiracial and ethnic, and issues that face lesbians across the age span.

Anne Figert
Associate Professor of Sociology
Loyola University Chicago

More pre-publication
REVIEWS, COMMENTARIES, EVALUATIONS . . .

What does it mean to be invisible? It means being denigrated or, worse, ignored. It means being silenced. Invisibility strips away the self, not with one swift, merciful pull, but slowly, painfully. Indeed, for the lesbians whose voices resonate throughout this book, invisibility may mean the difference between life and death. That is what is so important about this book: it renders the invisible glaringly visible. In *Gateways to Improving Lesbian Health and Health Care*, we hear lesbians recount their experiences in the health care system, a system in which providers assume every patient is straight and who privilege patients with white skin and well-stocked wallets. This book will make readers angry–angry enough, I hope, to do something about the injustice. Maybe a good place to start is getting this book into the hands of medical students and health care providers, forcing them to look in the mirror.

Claire M. Renzetti, PhD
Professor and Chair of Sociology, St. Joseph's University, Philadelphia, PA

Ponticelli's unprecedented collection goes to the source for powerful and poignant information on the state of lesbian health and health care. In stark contrast to most research, lesbians' own voices ring from the pages of these qualitative and quantitative studies on sexual abuse, domestic violence, aging, rural lesbians seeking local health care, and communicating with health care providers.

For years to come, this book will be seen as a gateway to the second generation of research on lesbian health and a milestone on the road to improving lesbian health and health care. This enlightening book is essential reading for all clinicians who care for lesbians and all researchers advancing the frontiers of lesbian health to meet the ever pressing needs.

Jocelyn C. White, MD, FACP, FAAPP
Assistant Professor of Medicine, Oregon Health Sciences University Faculty, Portland Program in General Internal Medicine, Legacy Portland Hospitals

Gateways to Improving Lesbian Health and Health Care: Opening Doors

∞ ALL HARRINGTON PARK PRESS BOOKS
ARE PRINTED ON CERTIFIED
ACID-FREE PAPER

Gateways to Improving Lesbian Health and Health Care: Opening Doors

Christy M. Ponticelli, PhD, MA, MTS
Editor

Gateways to Improving Lesbian Health and Health Care: Opening Doors, edited by Christy M. Ponticelli, was simultaneously issued by The Haworth Press, Inc., under the same title, as a special issue of the *Journal of Lesbian Studies,* Volume 2, Number 1, 1998, Esther D. Rothblum, Editor.

Harrington Park Press
An Imprint of
The Haworth Press, Inc.
New York • London

ISBN 1-56023-103-3

Published by

Harrington Park Press, 10 Alice Street, Binghamton, NY 13904-1580 USA

Harrington Park Press is an Imprint of the Haworth Press, Inc., 10 Alice Street, Binghamton, Ny 13904-1580 USA.

Gateways to Improving Lesbian Health and Health Care: Opening Doors has been co-published simultaneously as *Journal of Lesbian Studies*, Volume 2, Number 1 1998.

Cover design by Thomas J. Mayshock Jr.

Library of Congress Cataloging-in-Publication Data

Gateways to improving lesbian health and health care : opening doors / Christy M. Ponticelli, editor.
p. cm.
Includes bibliographical references and index.
ISBN 0-7890-0350-3 (alk. paper)–ISBN 1-56023-103-3 (alk. paper)
1. Lesbians–Health and hygiene. 2. Lesbians–Medical care. I. Ponticelli, Christy M.
RA564.87.G38 1998
362.1′086′643–dc21 97-30299
CIP

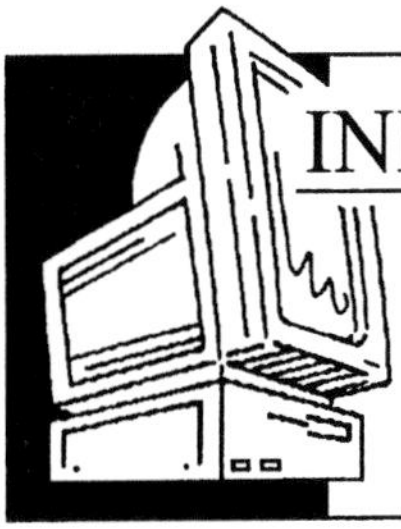

INDEXING & ABSTRACTING

Contributions to this publication are selectively indexed or abstracted in print, electronic, online, or CD-ROM version(s) of the reference tools and information services listed below. This list is current as of the copyright date of this publication. See the end of this section for additional notes.

- ***Abstracts in Social Gerontology: Current Literature on Aging,*** National Council on the Aging, Library, 409 Third Street SW, 2nd Floor, Washington, DC 20024
- ***CNPIEC Reference Guide: Chinese National Directory of Foreign Periodicals***, P.O. Box 88, Beijing, People's Republic of China
- ***Feminist Periodicals: A Current Listing of Contents,*** Women's Studies Librarian-at-Large, 728 State Street, 430 Memorial Library, Madison, WI 53706.
- ***Gay & Lesbian Abstracts,*** National Information Services Corporation, 306 East Baltimore Pike, 2nd Floor, Media, PA 19063
- ***HOMODOK/"Relevant" Bibliographic database, Documentation Centre for Gay & Lesbian Studies, University of Amsterdam (selective printed abstracts in "Homologie" and bibliographic computer databases covering cultural, historical, social and political aspects of gay & lesbian topics),*** HOMODOK-ILGA Archive, O.Z. Achterburgwal 185, NL-1012 DK Amsterdam, The Netherlands
- ***Index to Periodical Articles Related to Law,*** University of Texas, 727 East 26th Street, Austin, TX 78705
- ***INTERNET ACCESS (& additional networks) Bulletin Board for Libraries ("BUBL") coverage of information resources on INTERNET, JANET, and other networks.***
  - <URL:http://bubl.ac.uk/>
  - The new locations will be found under <URL:http://bubl.ac.uk/link/>.
  - Any existing BUBL users who have problems finding information on the new service should contact the BUBL help line by sending e-mail to <bubl@bubl.ac.uk>.

  The Andersonian Library, Curran Building, 101 St. James Road, Glasgow G4 0NS, Scotland

- ***Public Affairs Information Bulletin (PAIS),*** Public Affairs Information Service, Inc., 521 West 43rd Street, New York, NY 10036-4396
- ***Referativnyi Zhurnal (Abstracts Journal of the Institute of Scientific Information of the Republic of Russia),*** The Institute of Scientific Information, Baltijskaja ul., 14, Moscow, A-219, Republic of Russia
- ***Studies on Women Abstracts,*** Carfax Publishing Company, P.O. Box 25, Abingdon, Oxon OX14 3UE, United Kingdom
- ***Women's Studies Index (indexed comprehensively),*** G.K. Hall & Co., P.O. Box 159, Thorndike, ME 04986

SPECIAL BIBLIOGRAPHIC NOTES

related to special journal issues (separates) and indexing/abstracting

- ❑ indexing/abstracting services in this list will also cover material in any "separate" that is co-published simultaneously with Haworth's special thematic journal issue or DocuSerial. Indexing/abstracting usually covers material at the article/chapter level.
- ❑ monographic co-editions are intended for either non-subscribers or libraries which intend to purchase a second copy for their circulating collections.
- ❑ monographic co-editions are reported to all jobbers/wholesalers/approval plans. The source journal is listed as the "series" to assist the prevention of duplicate purchasing in the same manner utilized for books-in-series.
- ❑ to facilitate user/access services all indexing/abstracting services are encouraged to utilize the co-indexing entry note indicated at the bottom of the first page of each article/chapter/contribution.
- ❑ this is intended to assist a library user of any reference tool (whether print, electronic, online, or CD-ROM) to locate the monographic version if the library has purchased this version but not a subscription to the source journal.
- ❑ individual articles/chapters in any Haworth publication are also available through the Haworth Document Delivery Services (HDDS).

CONTENTS

ABOUT THE EDITOR

Christy M. Ponticelli, PhD, MA, MTS, is Assistant Professor of Sociology at the University of South Florida in Tampa. She holds degrees from Smith, Harvard Divinity and the University of California at Santa Cruz. Her research focuses on how the construction of homosexuality as a 'social problem' by dominant institutions, such as medicine and religion, affects gays and lesbians in their everyday realities. She is a reviewer for several sociology journals, and is Reviews Editor for the *Journal of Contemporary Ethnography.* Dr. Ponticelli is also a member of the American Sociological Association, the Society for the Study of Symbolic Interaction, and the Association for the Sociology of Religion.

Creating Awareness and Dialogue: Moving Toward Better Lesbian Health and Health Care

Christy M. Ponticelli

> How relevant are the *truths,* the experiences, the findings of white women to black women? Are women after all simply women?
>
> –Bambara (1970:9) [emphasis added]

It has been over two decades since Toni Cade Bambara asked these questions. Still, many institutions within our larger society have difficulty understanding women unless women assume a particular, stereotyped and mythical image of what is woman. Any person who represents or symbolizes a different image risks discrimination, oppression, dismissal or erasure. In the United States, our institution of health care, here broadly defined, is no model for understanding, even though it has demonstrated

---

Christy M. Ponticelli, PhD, MA, MTS, is currently Assistant Professor of Sociology at the University of South Florida where she teaches both undergraduate and graduate courses in Sexuality, Gender, Religion, Qualitative Methods, and Social Theory. Her research focuses on the construction of homosexuality as a social "problem," and on identity politics. She is currently the Reviews Editor for the *Journal of Contemporary Ethnography.*

Address correspondence to: Christy M. Ponticelli, Department of Sociology, University of South Florida, 4202 E. Fowler Avenue, CPR 107, Tampa, FL 33620-5550 (E-mail: ponticel@luna.cas.usf.edu).

[Haworth co-indexing entry note]: "Creating Awareness and Dialogue: Moving Toward Better Lesbian Health and Health Care." Ponticelli, Christy M. Co-published simultaneously in *Journal of Lesbian Studies* (The Haworth Press, Inc.) Vol. 2, No. 1, 1998, pp. 1-5; and: *Gateways to Improving Lesbian Health and Health Care: Opening Doors* (ed: Christy M. Ponticelli) The Haworth Press, Inc., 1998, pp. 1-5; and: *Gateways to Improving Lesbian Health and Health Care: Opening Doors* (ed: Christy M. Ponticelli) Harrington Park Press, an imprint of The Haworth Press, Inc., 1998, pp. 1-5. Single or multiple copies of this article are available for a fee from The Haworth Document Delivery Service [1-800-342-9678, 9:00 a.m. - 5:00 p.m. (EST). E-mail address: getinfo@haworth.com].

marked progress over the past fifty years. From the perspectives of lesbians, our health care institutions leave much to be desired.

First, there is the issue of finding a health care professional to whom we can openly discuss ourselves. Second, it is often difficult to find "adequate" care. Physician Katherine A. O'Hanlan offers evidence that demonstrates just how difficult it is to locate a health care practitioner who will or can treat lesbian patients with knowledgeable care. O'Hanlan (1995) surveyed 710 lesbian and gay doctors, 54% of whom reported that they had witnessed colleagues refuse to treat lesbians. In this same study, O'Hanlan surveyed lesbians (N = 13,543), discovering that lesbians in her study were less likely to receive routine screening tests (i.e., Pap smears, mammograms, or cholesterol screening) than heterosexual women, the comparison based on existing studies of heterosexual women. In some instances, lesbians were told by their physicians that they did not need these tests. Ironically, lesbians often have greater risk factors than heterosexual women when it comes to breast cancer (O'Hanlan 1995). In general, O'Hanlan found that many lesbians (72%) felt ostracized by their doctor, and 84% reported that they would not necessarily go back for treatment of new illnesses. These findings are not uncommon. In this collection of articles, for example, Tiemann, Kennedy and Haga report that one woman who came out as a lesbian to her physician was immediately referred to psychological treatment for her complaints. The woman later learned from another physician that she suffered from spinal compression.

What can be done to facilitate a better quality of health and health care for lesbians? In order to address this question, we need to know more about the everyday realities of self-identified lesbians, and the conditions that affect their health. What are experiences of lesbians as they attempt to identify and confront illness? What do lesbians consider "help," and where do they locate it? When they do seek help, what responses do they receive? By addressing these questions, we may begin to view experiences of lesbians less as isolated personal troubles and more as larger social issues (Mills 1959/1976). This, in turn, will help to analyze the construction of "lesbian" and "lesbianism" as a social problem within the health care arena (for more on the social problems work framework, see Miller and Holstein 1989, 1993; for a clear overview of the social construction of sexuality, see Weeks 1986). Only then can we hope to create a safer and healthier atmosphere for lesbians–in the larger society and in the specific locations where we seek to improve our health care.

To begin our exploration of lesbian health I start with three articles in which the authors go directly to the source for information. Lesbians are asked for their accounting of health-related issues. First, Joanne Hall asks lesbians who have survived childhood sexual abuse and are currently in alcohol misuse recovery programs to interpret their experiences. Hall draws her findings from 3 interviews each with 20 self-identified lesbians, 65% of whom are lesbians of color. Hall's study clearly substantiates the need to view sexualities as local histories and narratives (Plummer 1995; Weeks 1995).

Second, Teresa Scherzer explores domestic violence as experienced by lesbians in the San Francisco Bay area. Scherzer notes that hostility and discrimination often experienced by lesbians in everyday life pose additional challenges that heterosexuals ordinarily might not face. She states that this different social experience warrants research on lesbian domestic violence without comparing it to heterosexual domestic violence. While there is a growing body of literature addressing lesbian domestic violence (see Leeder 1988; Lie and Gentlewarrior 1991; Renzetti 1989, 1992), Scherzer's study focuses on psychological and emotional abuse, and includes a racially diverse sample with 44% of the respondents identifying as lesbians of color.

Third, lesbians' experiences with aging are explored by Barbara Herringer and Barbara Isaac, who highlight the general invisibility of aging lesbians in health and policy arenas. Herringer and Isaac note that while studies of the aging process are now emerging, what little we do know about women and aging is usually in comparison to what we know about men and aging. There is even less known about aging lesbians.

The last three articles in this collection address the more specific issue of direct contact between health care providers and lesbians. Each article offers insight into ways for improving this interaction. Kathleen Tiemann, Sally Kennedy and Myrna Haga focus on the strategies some rural lesbians use to come out to health care practitioners. Of particular difficulty to rural lesbians is the problem of finding information about potentially heterosexist or lesbian-friendly providers in a community that openly disapproves of difference.

Finally, Patricia Stevens, and Jocelyn White and Valerie Dull focus on what practitioners must do to assist in making health care more accessible to lesbians. Stevens offers a feminist narrative study, enabling lesbians of color to present personal accounts of prejudices they have encountered in face-to-face health care interactions. Her findings clearly demonstrate that health care practitioners must acknowledge and resolve their own prejudices, for the outcomes of not doing so pose grave dangers for those under their care. White and Dull, based on lesbians' perceptions of communication with medical and alternative primary care providers, argue that primary care providers must improve communication skills and attain a better knowledge base about sexual orientation in order to treat lesbian patients in a more sensitive and competent manner.

Certainly, one collection of articles cannot tell all that there is to know. But this collection can initiate an awareness, and hopefully a dialogue, about the "commonalities and differences" (Cole 1986) that exist for women in general, and lesbians in particular, regarding our health and the care that we receive. I hope that this publication generates greater awareness of health related issues within lesbian communities, but also within health care communities. Similarly, dialogue among lesbians and health care personnel is critical, but more importantly, I hope that these articles nurture dialogue between health care personnel and lesbians. Only by working together can we improve health care for lesbians.

In closing, I would like to thank the many individuals, from across disciplines, who assisted me with this publication by serving as anonymous reviewers. Peer reviewing is always a task, but these women and men, many of whom did not know me or the *Journal of Lesbian Studies*, went above and beyond in offering their professional assessment of articles submitted for this collection. I thank the following: George A. Appleby, Judith A. Baker, Evelyn Barbee, Karen Fox, Susan Krieger, Gwat-Yong Lie, Katherine A. O'Hanlan, Elizabeth Rankow, Brinda Rao, Claire Renzetti, Christine Saulnier, and Lynn S. Wilcox. Last but not least, I thank Diane, who has traveled through life with me, encouraging me at every step of the way, for over a decade now.

REFERENCES

Bambara, Toni Cade (Ed). (1970.) *The Black woman: An anthology.* New York: Signet.

Cole, Johnnetta B. (1986.) Commonalities and Differences. In J. Cole (Ed.) *All American women: Lines that divide, ties that bind* (pp. 1-30). New York: Free Press.

Hall, Joanne M. (1997.) Lesbians surviving childhood sexual abuse: Pivotal experiences related to sexual orientation, gender, and race. This volume.

Isaac, Barbara & Herringer, Barbara M. (1997.) Lesbian pass/ages: Invisible lives and issues of community. This volume.

Leeder, Elaine (1988.) Enmeshed in pain: Counseling the lesbian battering couple. *Women and Therapy,* 7(1), 81-99.

Lie, G.-Y., & Gentlewarrior, S. (1991.) Intimate violence in lesbian relationships: Discussion of survey findings and practice implications. *Journal of Social Service Research,* 15(1-2), 41-59.

Miller, Gale & Holstein, James A. (1989.) On the sociology of social problems. In J.A. Holstein & G. Miller (Ed.) in *Perspectives on social problems,* Vol. 1 (pp. 1-16) Greenwich, CT: JAI Press.

Miller, Gale, & Holstein, James A. (1993.) Social constructionism and social problems work. In G. Miller & J.A. Holstein (Ed.) *Constructionist controversies: Issues in social problems theory* (pp. 131-152) New York: Aldine de Gruyter.

Mills, C. Wright. (1959/1976.) *The sociological imagination*. New York: Oxford University Press.

O'Hanlan, Katherine A. (1995.) Lesbian health and homophobia: Perspectives for the treating obstetrician/gynecologist. *Current Problems in Obstetrics, Gynecology and Fertility,* 18(4), 97-127.

Plummer, Ken. (1995.) *Telling sexual stories*. New York: Routledge.

Renzetti, C.M. (1989.) "Building a second closet: Third party responses to victims of lesbian partner abuse. *Family Relations,* 38, 157-163.

Renzetti, C.M. (1992.) *Violent betrayal: Partner abuse in lesbian relationships*. Newbury Park, CA: Sage.

Scherzer, Teresa. (1997.) Domestic violence in lesbian relationships: Findings of the lesbian relationships research project." This volume.

Stevens, Patricia E. (1997.) Lesbians' of color experiences in health care encounters: Narrative insights for improving access and quality. This volume.

Tiemann, Kathleen A., Kennedy, Sally A. & Haga, Myrna P. (1997.) Rural lesbians' strategies for coming out to health care professionals." This volume.

Weeks, Jeffrey. (1986.) *Sexuality*. New York: Routledge.

Weeks, Jeffrey. (1995.) *Invented moralities: Sexual values in an age of uncertainty*. New York: Columbia University Press.

White, Jocelyn C., & Valerie T. Dull. (1997.) Room for improvement: Communication between lesbians and primary care providers. This volume.

Lesbians Surviving Childhood Sexual Abuse: Pivotal Experiences Related to Sexual Orientation, Gender, and Race

Joanne M. Hall

SUMMARY. This qualitative, feminist study is focused on lesbians' experiences growing up in multiproblem families, surviving afteref-

---

Joanne M. Hall, RN, PhD, is Associate Professor at University of Wisconsin-Milwaukee School of Nursing. She conducted the interviews for this research in 1993 and 1994 while she was a National Institutes of Health-supported Postdoctoral Fellow at University of California, San Francisco. She continues her focused life story research in Milwaukee with women recovering from alcohol problems who were sexually abused as children and is involved in intervention development for women who are dually affected by substance misuse and childhood sexual abuse. She has published widely related to lesbians and alcohol problems, childhood sexual abuse, women and work, nursing knowledge development, and feminist research methodologies and is a member of several editorial review boards of professional journals.

Address correspondence to: Joanne M. Hall, University of Wisconsin-Milwaukee, School of Nursing, P. O. Box 413, Milwaukee, WI 53201.

This research was funded through a National Research Service Award Individual Postdoctoral Fellowship from the National Institute of Nursing Research, National Institutes of Health #F32 NRO6817, sponsored by Afaf Ibrahim Meleis, PhD, F.A.A.N at University of California, San Francisco. The author acknowledges her colleagues at University of Wisconsin-Milwaukee, Jill Powell, RN, MSN, CS, and Patricia E. Stevens, RN, PhD, for their analytic assistance. The author is especially grateful to the women who shared their stories.

[Haworth co-indexing entry note]: "Lesbians Surviving Childhood Sexual Abuse: Pivotal Experiences Related to Sexual Orientation, Gender, and Race." Hall, Joanne M. Co-published simultaneously in *Journal of Lesbian Studies* (The Haworth Press, Inc.) Vol. 2, No. 1, 1998, pp. 7-28; and: *Gateways to Improving Lesbian Health and Health Care: Opening Doors* (ed: Christy M. Ponticelli) The Haworth Press, Inc., 1998, pp. 7-28; and: *Gateways to Improving Lesbian Health and Health Care: Opening Doors* (ed: Christy M. Ponticelli) Harrington Park Press, an imprint of The Haworth Press, Inc., 1998, pp. 7-28. Single or multiple copies of this article are available for a fee from The Haworth Document Delivery Service [1-800-342-9678, 9:00 a.m. - 5:00 p.m. (EST). E-mail address: getinfo@haworth.com].

fects of trauma, and struggling with alcohol problems. A multi-racial sample of 20 lesbians narrated life stories in a series of three in-depth interviews. The research report opens with one woman's narrative about surviving childhood sexual abuse and continues with explication of how differences and similarities within and between accounts pivot on the issues of sexual orientation, gender, and race. Results suggest that early in their lives, overwhelming violence and intrusive expectations were imposed, negating a clarity of experience about their authenticity. No participant expressed a belief that her sexual orientation was a result of childhood sexual abuse. The societal presumption of sexual abuse as an etiological factor in determining lesbian sexual orientation, nevertheless, was pivotal for these survivors because they had to constantly protect themselves from others' judgements about whether they were "real lesbians." They described a multi-faceted, ingenious strategy, gender-blurring, that helped them garner a place of some value in the family and stave off some of the violence, but this protective stance made them question whether they were "real women." Women also indicated that they grew up in families empty of cultural affiliation. Instead of knowledge and pride about connection with community, they experienced a gaping void about racial identification, ethnicity, parentage, and personal history. All in all, they survived a series of social identity exclusions. Conclusions call into question the usefulness and adequacy of theories about static psychological and social identities and suggest the importance of specific, localized analyses that explore narrative selves. *[Article copies available for a fee from The Haworth Document Delivery Service: 1-800-342-9678. E-mail address: getinfo@haworth.com]*

This qualitative, feminist study is focused on lesbians' experiences growing up in multiproblem families, surviving aftereffects of trauma, and struggling with alcohol problems. A multi-racial sample of 20 women who were recovering from alcohol problems and who also had histories of childhood sexual abuse narrated life stories in a series of three in-depth interviews. Specific research questions addressed in this paper are: (a) How do lesbians surviving childhood sexual abuse who are now in alcohol misuse recovery retrospectively interpret their experiences? (b) What differences and similarities within and between accounts pivot on the issues of sexual orientation, gender, and race? Results have the potential to fill gaps in knowledge about the aftereffects of childhood sexual abuse because most previous research has been unable to provide experiential detail specific to lesbians or women of color.

Aftereffects of childhood sexual abuse are disturbances in physical, mental, and relational health originating in or related to the trauma. Empirically documented aftereffects include: depression, low self-esteem, somatization, stress-associated illness, dissociation, post-traumatic stress disorder, distortions in self-image, anxiety, phobias, employment problems, impaired capacity for intimacy and sexual expression, parenting difficulties, and increased potential for revictimization in adulthood (Briere & Runtz, 1993; Fry, 1993; Hall, 1996b; Herman, 1992; Schetky, 1990; van der Kolk, McFarlane, & Weisaeth, 1996). Sexual abuse in childhood is also strongly associated with increased risk of substance misuse in adolescents and adult women. Likewise, women with substance misuse problems are more likely to report having been abused as children (Hurley, 1991). The type and duration of abuse, the child's age at onset, identity and number of perpetrators, degree of force used, occurrence of disclosure, and role of the child in the family constellation are all factors thought to influence the type and severity of aftereffects and have been well-researched (Browne & Finkelhor, 1986; Downs, 1993; Schetky, 1990).

Extant research, therefore, is informative about correlations among abuse characteristics and aftereffects, as well as prevalence. Epidemiological evidence suggests that one quarter of all females in the U.S. have experienced sexual abuse before age 18 (Finkelhor, Hotaling, Lewis, & Smith, 1990). What is missing from amassed quantitative data in the abuse literature is a well-articulated experiential perspective on surviving childhood sexual abuse from survivors' points of view. We also lack understanding of specific constraints to recovery, survival, and meaningful life posed for lesbians and women of color with histories of childhood sexual abuse. These subpopulations have not been adequately represented in research samples nor adequately described in research results (Hall, 1996a; 1996b).

METHODOLOGY

Sample

Inclusion criteria required participants to be at least 18 years old, self-identified as lesbian, self-identified as having an alcohol problem, abstinent from alcohol and other drugs for at least one year, and self-identified as a childhood sexual abuse survivor for at least one year. Participants were recruited through community-based purposive sampling (Biernacki & Waldorf, 1981). At the outset, research notices posted at lesbian gathering places and mailed to lesbian organizations exclusively invited the participation of lesbians of color who met inclusion criteria. Snowball sampling proceeded from initial interviews. After half of the sample had been recruited and interviewed, the study was opened to lesbians of all ethnic/racial backgrounds who met inclusion criteria. These steps assured ethnic/racial diversity among participants.

The sample was multi-racial as follows: 40% (8) African American, 35% (7) Euro-American, 15% (3) mixed race, and 10% (2) Latina. Ages ranged from 24 to 44; the mean was 34. The mean number of years of education was 13. This figure takes into account that 40% (8) of the women had dropped out of high school, most of whom later earned high school equivalency. Participants' incomes were low. The sample mean of $14,800 was only 42% of the average annual income in San Francisco (U.S. Department of Labor, 1994). Thirty-five percent (7) were unemployed; the rest worked in the service sector. Seventy percent (14) were in committed partnerships with other women at the time of the study. Thirty percent (6) had children.

All women in the study had been heavy drinkers. Almost all had been polydrug misusers. Generally, they had maintained long-term abstinence from alcohol and other drugs. The mean length of recovery was 4 years, ranging from 1 year to 10 years. All participants reported childhood sexual abuse categorized as severe or very severe, using Russell's (1986) criteria for severity: genital contact, long duration, and intrafamiliar and/or multiple perpetrators.

Data Collection

The design of the study consisted of focused life stories gathered over three separate interview sessions. Focused life stories is a retrospective qualitative design I adapted from life story methods (Bertaux & Kohli, 1984; Personal Narratives Group, 1989; Stivers, 1993) to elicit in-depth descriptions of life experiences about selected topics.

Data collection took place in San Francisco over several months in 1993 and 1994. Potential participants contacted me by telephone, I explained the study, and, as appropriate, we set an initial interview time and place. Interviews usually occurred in participants' homes or in my home. Upon meeting for each of the interviews, an informed consent process was followed as approved by the Committee on Human Research at University of California, San Francisco. At the end of the first and second interviews, subsequent interview appointments were set. Each interview lasted about two hours and was audiotaped. In addition to inquiring about alcohol use and recovery from alcohol problems, I asked open-ended questions about what it was like to grow up in their households, how they survived the abuse, and what it had meant to deal with its aftereffects in adulthood. I also inquired about their perspectives on how sociocultural identities (e.g., lesbian, woman, African American), might have affected their experiences. In field notes after interviews, I systematically documented nonverbal behaviors, power dynamics, context, rapport, interviewer and participant emotional responses, and flow of events (Briggs, 1986). All 20 participants completed the series of interviews, making for a total of 60 interviews. Participants earned a modest compensation of $20 for each interview.

Data Analysis

The 60 interviews were transcribed verbatim. To answer the research questions, I used a narrative analytic approach similar to one I developed in a previous feminist study of lesbians' alcohol problem recovery (Hall, 1994). I did successive readings of the 3 interview transcripts for each individual, systematically engaging in an exploration of a different type at each reading (Brown & Gilligan, 1992). First, I examined stories (Bell, 1988; Mishler, 1986; Polanyi, 1985; Riessman, 1993), diagramming story lines, dissecting plots, identifying operative actions, and scrutinizing participants' interpretations of events. I mapped associative links among stories told by individuals, and compared renderings of events across interview times. Another reading focused developmentally on the individual girl as she grew to adulthood, attending to how she negotiated the terrain of school-aged years and then adolescence and young adulthood shouldering the burden of severe abuse. A third analytic reading focused on how individuals integrated lesbian, gender, and ethnic/racial identifications. Then I compared narrative accounts across individuals searching for common experiences, perceptions, and beliefs among participants as well as what differentiated their stories from one another. At each stage, memos documented analytic insights. Throughout the process, I returned to the women's stories to evaluate the fit and appropriateness of developing analytic patterns (Josselson & Lieblich, 1995). Lastly, I examined life stories across the 20 participants once again to find an exemplar narrative account that illuminated analytic findings (Denzin, 1989). Adequacy of data collection and analysis were evaluated according to criteria of feminist rigor, including reflexivity, coherence, complexity, credibility, honesty, mutuality, and conscious partiality (Hall & Stevens, 1991).

RESULTS

Abbreviated Narrative Account

Vanessa's (pseudonym) story is one illustration of how lesbians surviving childhood sexual abuse and recovering from alcohol misuse retrospectively interpret their experiences. An abbreviated narrative account taken from her series of 3 interviews introduces the findings, providing a context for readers to understand what happened to participants. It is followed by description of narrative themes from the entire database and verbatim excerpts from a range of participants' accounts. To authentically convey the stories women told about their lives, some degree of explicit detail about traumatic events is necessary.

Vanessa, a 24 year old African-American lesbian, was sexually and physically abused and neglected as a child. Her mother and biological father divorced when Vanessa was 4 years old. She grew up in a chaotic home where her mother, diabetic and addicted to heroin, allowed boyfriends and drug customers to come and go. At the outset of the first interview, Vanessa said she was not sure if she qualified for the study because, although she had been abused, others had surely had worse experiences. She said maybe hers "wasn't that bad":

> I remember being weird. I wasn't like the rest of the kids. They didn't have to worry about–do you think Mom has passed out? Is she in a coma? Is there food in the house? I had a lot of responsibilities–I started cooking when I was 6 yrs old. I had to make sure my sister and I had our clothes for school. And hopefully Mom don't die while we are at school. With her diabetes, plus she was a heroin and speedball user, she might OD and I had to be aware of that. If people came into the house, I always had to watch to see if they were stealing something. . . . My mother would have me hold all the money. I'd go to school with hundreds and hundreds of dollars, and I would have to be responsible for this money, so that we could have things. I had to grow up real quick. And because I was like a grown-up, I think what happened was that grown men were attracted to me.
>
> When my Mom got divorced, she worked. And during that time was my first abuse. This babysitter would–he wouldn't physically abuse me–but–oh yes, he would physically abuse me. He would tell me to go look at the stars at night and tell him what I saw. And I would say, "I see the stars and the moon," and he would whip my ass. He would whip my ass until I'd pass out. And that's all I remember. I never understood. And I was scared because he said if I told, he would kill my Mom. After a while, my Mom started realizing that my sister and me never wanted her to leave. She finally sat me down and I told her. She got rid of him.
>
> I learned how to masturbate, but it was just to relieve the pain, a pain that I felt down there. I learned how to relieve that pain; it

wasn't like an orgasm. But my grandmother used to talk about me real bad. She caught me and called me all kinds of names like slut and stuff.

As a tot I drank whatever was left in the glasses. My Mom thought it was cute, but I would be getting drunk. My grandmother used to yell at me for drinking her beer. I was basically the black sheep. Vanessa, the liar and the thief. I did steal, because I didn't have anything.

You know those books about families with vacations and fathers and meals and all that? This was not my house. I would come home and find junkies falling out that I had to step over. And no food. Other little kids were playing hopscotch and jacks. I'm worried about what's happening at home. Is my Mom ok? Her addiction was rough. She wouldn't be able to pay the rent, so we moved a lot. High school was the first time I was able to go the whole 4 years in one school. I was still the outcast. I hooked up with this female that I was attracted to, but not knowing that I was attracted. We smoked weed. We would get so drunk. Whatever anybody had, we would try it.

After high school, I realized I liked women. I had my first reality of *knowing* that I was having sex with a woman. Now, I understand why I didn't really relate to other guys, the sexual thing, nothing was there. When I came out, that's when freebasing came out. So that was just the next step. I lost my job. I graduated to smoking crack, and then to shooting speed and crank. I tried heroin. I wanted to know what Mom was feeling. I liked crank. It would make me forget about any kind of problems I had. I'd get up and be laughing, the world would be great, and I'd clean my house–the walls, every drawer, fold everything, clean the outside of the drawers. I could block out those sexual abuse things. They just weren't there. I didn't think about them. But, when I wasn't high, I would remember the times I had been raped . . .

My Mom was a very kind-hearted person. Somebody would say, "I don't have a place" and she'd say, "You can sleep on the couch." And they'd be in the house. This one guy beat my sister, and he pulled me in the bathroom and raped me and then beat me. He made me have sex with him. My Mom said that I was in shock. They had to take me to the hospital. My Mom had to tell me; I didn't remember. All I remember was this man coming into the house and my sister and me trying to pretend that we were asleep–but we weren't. And he took me in the bathroom. In the hospital, I got real scared because the doctor started touching me down there. I was in the second grade.

We would go spend the summer with my father. His new wife had two sons. I remember my step-brother getting on top of me, and I was scared. He said that he would beat me up if I told. I didn't tell for quite some time. And he would have sex with me. I still haven't told his mother. It started when I was about 7 and kept up until I was about 13 or 14. He must have told his other brother, because he did it, too.

Then there was this guy who was keeping my Mom high. One of the things he did was he made me and my sister take some pills. And I remember being in this bathtub and he put oil on us and took these naked porno pictures. So there are pictures of us being handed around somewhere. I had a lot of–those kinds of things happen to me before I was even 10 . . .

Abandonment was a big part of what was happening to me as I grew up. My Mom would go out, make a connection, get arrested, and not come back. My sister and me might be in the house for 2 or 3 days with nobody there. So, today, I wind up clinging to people in relationships. While I was using, I had sex with so many guys, I thought that I'd never be able to enjoy sex again. It's like I had a real deep hole of loneliness going through me–I was very sad.

I still have trouble and I'm not taking care of myself too good right now. I forget about my recovery program, my friends. I shut down. I tried to be what my last girlfriend wanted me to be–and not be me. I tried therapy. I got my girlfriend to go to the therapy, but she didn't want to participate. So I decided to just keep going alone. But the lady didn't know anything about lesbian relationships. Relationships with women are a little bit more intense–for me, anyway. Like you and that other person against the majority of the world. You go through a lot of persecution because of that. The lady didn't get it. It was terrible, like talking to a wall. She was just agreeing with everything I was saying.

It didn't work out with my last girlfriend because she wanted me to be more fem. She said I could wear jeans, but they had to be bought in the ladies section. I didn't like that, and they didn't fit me, anyway. She wanted to buy me earrings and I said I wanted the posts, just the gold stud kind. She got gold rings. I hated them. I didn't feel right in them. I have to have that balance. She thought it was no big deal. But it was for me. . . . So for now, I am not having relationships.

Why I cling so much to my friends and my lovers is that I don't trust that much and I feel any problem is always my fault. Because of

> sexual abuse I have phobias, like getting hugs in recovery. If you hug me too long it's like–ugh. Just let me go. DON'T TOUCH ME!

Suddenly in the middle of her narration, Vanessa stared wide-eyed at me, as if just remembering something very frightening. She blurted out:

> I HAD GOT RAPED BY THIS GUY ON THE STREET. And I was screaming for help–I was screaming–and these people closed their windows and others walked by. I got beat up really bad–real bad. I went to the doctor and he said I was all torn up inside. And my friends didn't BELIEVE me. That reminds me of something else. Getting drunk over at a friend's house, and when I woke up I was being gang raped. I had no choice, and I didn't even know how long they had been doing it.
>
> Ain't nobody gonna believe me anyway. I'm just a liar and a thief and nobody is gonna believe me. My Mom didn't believe me all those times because these men were giving us gifts and getting her high. I had to be the strong one. I was so little, but it was my job to get the dangerous guys out of my Mom's house. You turn off the fear and then you just go ahead and do it. I had to threaten these two hundred pound guys that I'd kill them or get someone else to cut them up . . .

Narrative Themes

Many themes of Vanessa's account were echoed in other women's narratives, demonstrating how pivotal sexual orientation, gender, and race were in their lives. An elaboration of six narrative themes synthesized from the analysis of their stories of surviving childhood sexual abuse and recovering from alcohol problems follow.

Never a child. A clear theme in Vanessa's story was the role reversal often seen in families where abuse occurs. Vanessa was "parentified" early on, and was painfully aware of not having the apparently carefree life she saw in glimpses of schoolmates' experiences. Though she had been sexualized by adults in her preschool years, including sadistic whipping, she lamented that no one had ever really educated her about sex. She was an adult before she recognized what an orgasm was. *All participants described feeling "robbed" of a childhood regardless of the age of onset, duration, or type of abuse they suffered.* They were forced to meet adults' needs in adult ways before they could recognize or trust their own childhood experiences. The self-image of never having been innocent was deeply ingrained, and the source of significant distress. Many spoke of having to "pay for everything," especially for attention and "love." One woman said that during her early school-aged years, the exchanges of sex for candy and money gave her the illusion of being powerful. But as an adult she felt "ripped off, shoved into the dirt, never to have felt pure and clean."

Questioning abuse. All woman in this study could be considered severely abused by the most conservative standards, and each had clear memories of multiple perpetrations. Their narrations were remarkable, however, in that they repeatedly applied qualifications to their descriptions, discounting the importance and severity of their abuse, blaming themselves for somehow causing the violations. Like Vanessa, many participants worried that they were not "qualified" to be in the study. Having ever been given bribes or pacification with candy, alcohol, food, or money in conjunction with abuse episodes was a disqualifying factor in some women's minds. Others concluded that if a bodily sensation in response to a sexual act was ever experienced, it must not have really been abuse. If perpetrators were "just brothers," it was probably "kid's play"; even if the brother was 14 and the sister was 3. If the participant did not tell anyone about it, she might present the abuse as her own fault, despite the death threats she experienced. If one was a lesbian, or a "tomboy," perhaps outgoing, physical play may have "tempted" adults into the sexual situation. Survivors' doubts about the reality and severity of sexual abuse were not only apparent in accounts of privatized, secretive violence, and dissociated memories; but were also apparent in accounts wherein witnesses to the abuse were present, crimes were discovered in *flagrant delicto,* and perpetrators admitted their guilt. Overall, the sense of their own legitimacy as abuse survivors was tenuous, almost no matter the context.

"True lesbianism." All participants were asked their perspective on how being lesbian might have affected their experiences. Some participants had logical responses, philosophizing about how there seemed to be a disproportionate number of lesbian survivors of sexual abuse. They wondered if there was a connection between the two factors, but were not certain what that might be. A few mused that perhaps abused lesbians gravitate to each other in mutual support, creating the impression for lesbians that they are abused more often than heterosexual women. Others said that they knew equal numbers of heterosexual women who were sexually abused. A few said that lesbians were not disproportionately abused, but might more often *disclose* abuse. They reasoned that lesbians typically do not depend on men economically, and therefore can be more critical of male perpetrators.

Most participants went on to respond emotionally, however, describing how their histories of sexual abuse in childhood made them apprehensive about their authenticity as lesbians. This questioning of their "true lesbianism" took many forms. Only two participants said that they worried that victimization by males may have "made women seem more attractive" to them:

- I guess if I got all that abuse from men, it could figure in to my being lesbian. But then my mother was probably more damaging to me. She said I was ugly and dumb. And she hit me all the time. It is a wonder I trust women at all. So I must be gay if I still seek out women in spite of my mother's abuse. I don't know. Am I looking for a mother to love me? I have always found women more attractive than men.
- The sexual abuse I got was from men. So, no, I don't think they would hold a lot of attraction for me. Is being lesbian caused by anything? The way I was ignored by my mother would have made me *seek men* for attention. So that wouldn't be logical. What causes heterosexual women who are abused by their fathers to still be attracted to men?

Essentially all participants rejected direct causal connection between sexual orientation and sexual abuse:

- Are you asking do I think I am a lesbian because I was abused? No. They are not related. Incest by my uncle and my brother was not sexuality. It was violence, brutality against a child. I remember becoming an adolescent and feeling turned on to see the girls undress in gym. It was natural for me. I didn't understand it all completely then, but when other girls were giggling about their boyfriends, I was fantasizing about my best girlfriend.
- I probably could sexually relate to a man or a woman. But I find that most men don't reach my basic criteria for relationships: commitment and emotional honesty. I think abuse has made me wary of everybody, male or female. But when I have had sex with women, it is clear to me that it is more pleasing to me. I am woman-focused, a lesbian. And no, you don't become a lesbian because somebody raped you.

But, women worried that others would mistakenly conclude that childhood sexual abuse had "caused" their lesbianism:

- As far as I can remember, I have felt attracted to women. But I'm careful when I talk to people about being sexually abused, because I don't want it to feed the Freudian stereotypes. Like if a man hurts you, you turn to women as a second choice. I was definitely lesbian from the start.

- I don't believe my being a lesbian is a result of being abused. It is too much a core part of me to be the result of any *one* thing. I feel the abuse experiences and being a lesbian are separate, but being a lesbian does make my recovery more complicated. I don't tell people I am a lesbian who was sexually abused as a kid, because I don't want them to jump to the wrong conclusion, like a bad stereotype.

Women described making many efforts to protect themselves against the pathologizing "stereotype" that sexual abuse causes lesbianism. They lived in anticipation of others' presumptions and thus felt challenge to the authenticity of their sexual orientation. As one woman put it:

- I am unsure, and can never really quite be certain if I am a *real lesbian* because my sexual development was screwed up so early in my life.

The issue of who are "real lesbians" has been debated about woman who identify as lesbians later in life, lesbians who have sex with men, celibate lesbians, women of color who have sex with women but do not call themselves lesbians, etc. These debates about identity are of little comfort, however, to women who feel that the abuse they survived has made them markedly different from other lesbians:

- I can listen to women when they talk about lesbian oppression, and how their families didn't accept them about this, or even those who have gotten eventual affirmation from their families. But I don't see that the discrimination against lesbians has damaged me as much as the abuse has. And I am not in any hurry to reconcile with my family. What I need is to stay away from those people.

Many participants differentiated themselves as not "fitting in" with the "lesbian community." If lesbians are defined by their sexual behavior, that is, as women who have sex with other women and who form sexually based coupled relationships with each other, then sexual abuse survivors are "anomalies." Like Vanessa, many women in this study had great difficulty with trust, intimacy, and sexual relating because of their histories of sexual abuse. Many were alienated or frightened by commonly accepted activities like "sexual banter" at lesbian gatherings:

- I went to a party, and I just wore sweats, nothing dressed up. And I had this woman touch my arm and come up with this stuff about "how attractive I was this evening." I was furious. And then when there was all this talk about butch and fem and sexual stuff, I wanted out of there. It is too much. I got my partner and said, I gotta go home. *Now.* She didn't quite understand, but she went home with me. These lesbian groups think it is fine, like liberating, to bring up that sexual stuff, and fantasies, but they have no idea how it affects some people. It is not liberating for me.
- I have sometimes felt when I walked into a lesbian AA (Alcoholics Anonymous) meeting that it was a meat market. Women looking you up and down. I come there to get sober and here are these flirtations going on. It's much more serious with me. I don't expect someone coming on to me there. I can get that in a bar.

Lacking a sense of belonging in social situations and feeling threatened in interpersonal relations with other lesbians, participants were reinforced in their doubts about the "truth" of their lesbianism.

Gender-blurring. Most participants related having adopted a "gender-blurred" approach to life. During childhood and adolescence, participants perceived that by behaving as a boy they might: (a) mend multi-problem families, (b) gain parental love, (c) fulfill a male sexual role with a female abuse perpetrator, (d) affiliate non-sexually with "protective" male peers, and/or (e) avoid "feminine attractiveness" that could bring danger.

Participants' stories revealed how this gender-blurring happened. In early childhood, "tomboy" behavior was often a response to an expectation, for instance, that they protect mothers who were depressed, addicted, or alone. Many served as "eldest sons," "big brothers" to younger siblings, decision-makers, and liaisons to the "outside world" for inept families that were closed, secretive, and neglectful. Some received clear messages, spoken and unspoken, that their parents had wanted a son. In trying to gain their love and approval, the girl child had to play the "little boy." A few had mothers or other adult females who were sexual abuse perpetrators. This, too, often encouraged the child to act in "male ways." Some were able, at least for some segments of their childhoods, to fit into male social circles in their neighborhoods as one of the "guys," acting as a "buddy" or "mascot." Many described a period in their early adolescence when, unlike their peers, they adopted baggy jeans and T-shirts, and wore no makeup in order to avoid appearing female. It was unsafe to be a woman; a woman was "weak" and "vulnerable." This avenue of self-protection from danger was less available to girls who quickly developed large breasts and a "pear" or "hour-glass" physique.

Socializing with and appearing to be the opposite gender may have been an attempt to dissuade male perpetrators from victimizing them, but it did not save them from the merciless criticism, usually from mothers, about their non-conformity to traditional gender role expectations. Note that in her narrative, Vanessa refers to not having sex with "other guys," a possible indication of the gender-blurring she experienced and simultaneously had to create in her life. Even as a little girl, she had to act the "man of the house," fending off male intruders, protecting her mother, managing the money. Common across stories of gender-blurring was its strategic value. Gender-blurring was not an identity issue per se. Most of the time, for these women, the strategy was to *avoid being female* so as to camouflage themselves against potential abuse. In a society that has narrowly defined its gender roles via appearance and behavior and has prioritized male identity, this strategy is possible; because to *not act like a girl* will appear, by default, as *being a boy.* Participants' self-protective behaviors along these lines cannot be taken, therefore, to mean they believed themselves to be of the opposite sex.

- I did not shave my underarms, and when, one day on the bus, I put my arms back to rest my head, a boy came by and said, "Ugh, look how hairy you are." I am not, you know, pretty. I didn't want to wear dresses. I wore a flannel shirt, and hung out with the boys in the street when I still lived in Mexico. We would drink every night, and they protected me. Only a few times they excluded me. But mostly I was accepted in the group.
- I can still pass, and often do, for a young black male. I like being able to fool people, because I'm safe then. I lived as a boy for nine months during my sixteenth year. I would change my clothes outside after I left the house every morning and change back every evening when I had to go home. In high school, my girlfriend wanted me to have a sex change operation. . . . But, I didn't actually want to *be* a man. . . . Now my recovery is about using music to allow my feminine self to come out.

Indeed, participants who, at times, used their androgynous qualities to appear male/masculine were not attempting to become male. Prior experience had set them up for a dilemma in which being identifiably female/feminine was dangerous. Actions to be safe (i.e., to not be a girl), nevertheless derailed their certainty and comfort with "femaleness" and contributed to doubts that they were "real women." Gender-blurring marked their experience of *being a woman* as quite different from what they believed the majority experience was.

Cultural void. Participants' stories revealed childhood homes void of cultural identification and pride. The fact that abuse and covert sexual violence were going on within families was evidently not all that was kept secret. As girls, several of the participants had not known who their biological fathers were, did not know their exact date of birth, and lacked knowledge of ethnic/racial heritage. Some homes were run by strict, physically punitive religious standards, yet girls did not know of any affiliation with a church denomination.

Striking findings were discovered in responses to a demographic query, How do you describe yourself racially and ethnically? Some women were angry at being asked, as though their *skin color* was apparent and no further distinctions could be made. For instance, one African American-appearing woman stated she "did not see color," then looked at her skin and said she guessed she was "brown." Musing aloud about what color her friends were, she said she thought they were "pink." Later in the same interview, she described agonizing isolation in being the only Black student in an all White school when she was growing up. She related that in those same years when she was a pre-teen, she suffered nightly sexual abuse by brothers who broke into her room. After each of these attacks, she would shower and rub chlorine bleach into her skin. For her, this action seemed to have implications about the shame she felt about the sexual violation as well as the pain endured because of her dark skin color.

Most participants stumbled and hesitated in response to the question about their ethnic/racial identification:

- I am White. I don't know. I don't have any ethnicity that I know of.
- I guess I would say White. My parents never mentioned it.
- Black. I don't go for that Afro-American stuff. I know there is some kind of African culture, but I don't know anything about it. I know there was slavery. That's it.

Some described their pain and confusion:

- I didn't fit in anywhere. I am half Cuban and half Irish. My folks were ashamed of this and so I think they just let me think I was White. When I got to school, I was shocked. I was called nigger and spic. Then when I tried to join up with groups, I was rejected. I wasn't really Black, not really Latina, as far as they were concerned. And my one White friend, she told me that her mother had forbidden her to ever bring me home with her.

In subsequent interviews, these same women often described a longing to have some information about their cultural heritage, believing it would aid in their recovery process:

- It would help if I knew more about African-American history. I could feel proud. I am not too proud of my own family. They are all dope fiends. . . . I know about scamming, but not about my own people.
- I am claiming my father's Native American culture, even though he does not acknowledge his tribe. I go to the talking circles and sweat lodges for recovery. I am half Filipino. I am both. Both cultures are important to me now.

For a small sub-sample in the study, cultural tradition had significant, direct influence on their interpretations of sexual abuse in childhood, but not for the good. Latina participants who were raised in strict Catholic homes and schools understood as girls that vaginal penetration meant loss of virginity. Unable to make a distinction about the fact that this was done against their will, they felt like damaged goods. Even if they were conscious of being lesbians, not planning heterosexual marriage, the loss of virginity still carried its basic message: No one will want you. They often reacted by becoming, in their words, "promiscuous" with many male sexual partners.

Targeting. The women often talked about being "marked" for abuse. Many believed they became objects targeted by perpetrators because of their racial features, resemblance to a hated other, and/or identification as a lesbian. Mixed race women, in particular, recalled scapegoating incidents related to skin color. In the case of one participant, the darker-skinned elder children in the family were referred to as "cousins" and became family servants. This woman recounted finding out at age 21 that the household "maids" in her childhood home were actually her half-sisters. In several families, mothers had a series of marriages and children from each, moving to lighter and lighter-skinned husbands with each partnership.

The denigration of darker skin hues was also experienced by participants in their mothers' insistence that they never marry a Black or Mexican man. One woman, who had darker features than any of her siblings, grew up verbally abused by her Euro-American mother and sexually abused by her Middle Eastern father. In her early adolescence, her father left the family. She was harangued by her mother to "marry a White man," and in defiance, ran away as a teen with a Black man. She was "turned out" by him as his prostitute. Subsequently, he impregnated her.

She was able to escape back to her mother's home only to be met with furious rage. The mother ignored and mistreated the mixed race grandchild. Tragically, this participant's son disappeared at age 3, leaving her grief-stricken for many years. She was plagued by questions about whether her son might still be with her if her mother had been willing to help care for him as she did the White grandchildren.

There were several women who were quite certain that it was both skin color and resemblance to estranged biological fathers that left them unprotected and targeted in the family. For example, one woman was sexually abused in childhood by her mother. This participant was, like her biological father, a fair-skinned Latino. The sexual abuse seemed to be the mother's way of contacting her lost lover through the child who resembled him, and an expression of anger at his abandonment of her. In another example, an African American participant said:

- My mother screamed all the time about how I looked like my no-good father. My hair was too nappy. She would call my sister her "golden baby," because she was lighter and born at a time when my mother had good business. I begged other relatives to take me in. Of course, when I was abused by men that my mother let in the house, I was so starved for love, I would feel special and cared for by them. I had no framework for seeing this attention as abuse then.

The pain these girls were subjected to by virtue of their racially-based physical characteristics had ramifications outside the home. Many women of color recalled being excluded from almost every social group in school, except perhaps the drug-using group. An immigrant Latina told the story of having developed a fixation on a blonde, blue-eyed, popular girl in her high school class. She stared at her every day for a year, even though the two never met or spoke. It seemed as if the Latina girl was experiencing a sexual attraction to the fair, White girl. In addition, she harbored the belief that, "If I was her, this [sexual abuse as a child and later adolescent rape] would never have happened to me."

Lesbian-associated behavior or affiliation could also mark girls for sexual abuse. Several women of color in the study perceived that being "gay" targeted them:

- Yeah, when I was a kid, I was this little tomboy romping all over. I think maybe it made me a target, either to get me in line, or because my physical activity got mistaken for something else. Or is it just that I think everything is my fault because it happened to me? Who knows?

These women recounted stories of risking violence and having unwanted sex with men to preserve their sexual and social inclinations toward females:

- When we were in middle school, us gay girls hung together. In my neighborhood, you didn't want to be caught alone. The guys would pull the train (gang-rape) on a girl if they thought she was a lezzie.
- As an African-American, I didn't want to be known as a dyke. Some guys look for dykes to rape, basically. Or they constantly come at you. Like "You just haven't had it done right, by a real man." I would periodically have sex with a guy, to get everybody off my back. Now I wouldn't do that. I realize that every time I have let somebody use my body it has done me damage in my soul.

CONCLUSIONS

In this qualitative study, a multi-racial sample of 20 lesbians recovering from alcohol problems who had histories of childhood sexual abuse narrated life stories in a series of three in-depth interviews. In their accounts they described growing up in multiproblem families, surviving aftereffects of trauma, and struggling with alcohol problems. A major thread in these women's accounts was the sense that they had fallen short of what is necessary to be a "real" person. The central contradictory experience was never being allowed to be a child. Early in their lives, overwhelming violence and intrusive expectations were imposed, negating a clarity of experience about their "authenticity." In growing up, the abuse and its aftermath marked the self as "not belonging" anywhere. They tended to doubt whether they were "real" sexual abuse survivors because they didn't think the horrors they survived were worse than those of others, or because minimization was a defense they needed to function day to day.

No participant expressed a belief that her sexual orientation was a result of childhood sexual abuse. The societal presumption of sexual abuse as an etiological factor in determining lesbian sexual orientation, nevertheless, was pivotal for these survivors because it was only a step away from the possible conclusion that one is not a lesbian at all, but merely living out the script of an abused person avoiding reminders of the past. The ideology that lesbianism is a product of incest was a constituent of pathologizing theories purported throughout the century by "medical authorities" who equated lesbian identity with sickness and evil (Stevens & Hall, 1991). Such theories have had profound effect on public opinion and sentiment toward lesbians. The women in this study described constantly protecting themselves from others' presumptions and thus they felt challenge to the authenticity of their sexual orientation. There was also varying intensity of doubt about being a "real lesbian" if, because of the aftereffects of sexual abuse, one had difficulty engaging in intimate contact with other women, or felt unsafe or alienated in lesbian gatherings.

The multi-faceted, ingenious protective strategy these lesbians employed from early childhood, gender-blurring, helped them garner a place of some value in the family and stave off some of the violence. They used their androgynous qualities to appear male/masculine, not because they identified as male, but because they yearned to be loved and to be safe. Their abuse experiences had set them up for a dilemma in which being identifiably female/feminine was dangerous. Hence, ability to be "one of the guys," discomfort with feminine attire, and fear of sexual banter and flirting were all protective measures. But, these aspects of their daily lives made some women doubt their authenticity as "real women." Women also indicated that one is not a "real person" if one has no cultural heritage. Participants grew up in families empty of affiliation. Instead of knowledge and pride about connection with community, they experienced a gaping void about racial identification, ethnicity, parentage, and personal history.

One might venture that because of the first invalidation, that of being a child, the other insults to authenticity followed, toppling one's certainty in each identity like dominoes. It is much easier to find proof of exclusion from a category or group than to ensure inclusion. One shaky brick in the foundation is often enough to create the perception that one "does not belong." When the initial sense of one's self as real, as a child safely doing what children are capable of doing, is jerked away, the stage is set for invalidation on nearly all fronts. These women were not permitted childhoods because, in their young years, ghastly violence, adult sexuality, and character annihilation were thrust into their bodies and souls. They were "robbed" of safety and protection from trustworthy adults, innocent play and exploration, free and easy unfolding of sexual orientation, and unfettered "trying on" of gender roles. Rootedness that should have come from cultural affiliation was either non-existent in their childhood homes or twisted into a mark of vulnerability. These findings underscore the depth of alienation, struggle, and abandonment experienced by these women. More questions must be answered. How do women like those in this study survive the series of social identity exclusions they experienced? How much energy is daily expended in nurturing fragile threads of connection with others? How do they balance damaging emotional propaganda about their many counts of illegitimacy with the realities of what they had to do to survive abuse?

The experiences of these women call into question theories that rely on immutable qualities of identity. Consistent with recent articulations countering the usefulness and adequacy of static psychological and social identities (Haraway, 1991; Phelan, 1994; Stone, 1996), findings of this study demonstrate the complexity of women's lives and suggest the importance of specific, localized analyses that claim the irreducibility of persons to categories (Phelan, 1994; Probyn, 1996). Inquiry predicated on strict categorization of sexual orientation, gender, and race is not coherent with the passage of human experience and its imprint upon narrative selves.

The sense of inauthenticity or falseness experienced by these lesbians surviving childhood sexual abuse is not merely an internal psychological aftereffect of having been abused, or even of being multiply stigmatized. At almost every turn in their attempts to survive and recover, they felt, and indeed were questioned, as to their legitimacy as lesbians, women, and members of specific ethnic/racial groups. They had to proceed from major blows to their existence in childhood and grow up in day-to-day struggle with a society that demands that people "stay put" within their respective social boxes, whether these boxes are lined with velvet or barbed wire. In the study of women's lives, the concept of identity may be less meaningful than we had previously thought, and may actually further the damage suffered if integrity is predicated on the categories one fits instead of on the sojourn one has traveled.

In this study, I was able to access only women survivors of childhood sexual abuse who were able to tell their stories. Others have met death by addiction, suicide, or homicide at the hands of an abuser. Many more are terrified into secrecy, amnesia, or mental illness by the aftermath of childhood abuse. The battle for women's lives must continue in their honor.

REFERENCES

Bell, S. E. (1988). Becoming a political woman: The reconstruction and interpretation of experience through stories. In A. D. Todd & S. Fisher (Eds.), *Gender and discourse: The power of talk* (pp. 97-123). Norwood, NJ: Ablex.

Bertaux, D. & Kohli, M. (1984). The life story approach: A continental view. *Annual Review of Sociology, 10,* 215-237.

Biernacki, P., & Waldorf, D. (1981). Snowball sampling: Problems and techniques of chain referral sampling. *Sociological Methods and Research, 10,* 141-163.

Briere, J., & Runtz, M. (1993). Childhood sexual abuse: Implications for psychological assessment. *Journal of Interpersonal Violence, 8*(3), 312-330.

Briggs, C. L. (1986). *Learning how to ask: A sociolinguistic appraisal of the role of the interview in social science research.* New York: Cambridge University Press.

Brown, L. M., & Gilligan, C. (1992). *Meeting at the crossroads: Women's psychology and girls' development.* Cambridge, MA: Harvard University Press.

Browne, A., & Finkelhor, D. (1986). Impact of child sexual abuse: A review of the research. *Psychological Bulletin, 99,* 66-77.

Denzin, N. K. (1989). *Interpretive interactionism.* Newbury Park, CA: Sage.

Downs, W. R. (1993). Developmental considerations for the effects of childhood sexual abuse. *Journal of Interpersonal Violence, 8*(3), 331-345.

Finkelhor, D., Hotaling, G., Lewis, I., & Smith, C. (1990). Sexual abuse in a national survey of adult men and women: Prevalence, characteristics and risk factors. *Child Abuse and Neglect, 14*(1), 19-28.

Fry, R. (1993). Adult physical illness and childhood sexual abuse. *Journal of Psychosomatic Research, 37*(2), 89-103.

Hall, J. M. (1994). How lesbians recognize and respond to alcohol problems: A theoretical model of problematization. *Advances in Nursing Science, 16*(3), 46-63.

Hall, J. M. (1996a). Geography of childhood sexual abuse: Women's narratives of their childhood environments. *Advances in Nursing Science, 18*(4), 29-47.

Hall, J. M. (1996b). The pervasive effects of childhood sexual abuse in lesbians' recovery from alcohol problems. *Substance Use and Misuse, 31*(2), 225-239.

Hall, J. M., & Stevens, P. E. (1991). Rigor in feminist research. *Advances in Nursing Science, 13*(3), 16-29.

Haraway, D. (1991). *Simians, cyborgs and women: The reinvention of nature.* New York: Routledge.

Herman, J. L. (1992). *Trauma and recovery.* New York: Basic Books.

Hurley, D. L. (1991). Women, alcohol, and incest: An analytical review. *Journal of Studies on Alcohol, 52*(3), 253-268.

Josselson, R., & Lieblich, A. (Eds.). (1995). *Interpreting experience [The narrative study of lives]* (Vol. 3). Thousand Oaks, CA: Sage.

Mishler, E. G. (1986). *Research interviewing: Context and narrative.* Cambridge, MA: Harvard University Press.

Personal Narratives Group (Eds.). (1989). *Interpreting women's lives: Feminist theory and personal narratives.* Bloomington, IN: Indiana University Press.

Phelan, S. (1994). *Getting specific: Postmodern lesbian politics.* Minneapolis: University of Minnesota Press.

Polanyi, L. (1985). *Telling the American story: A structural and cultural analysis of conversational storytelling.* Norwood, NJ: Ablex.

Probyn, E. (1996). *Outside belongings.* New York: Routledge.

Putnam, F. W. (1990). Disturbances of "self" in victims of child sexual abuse. In R. P. Kluft (Ed.), *Incest-related syndromes of adult psychopathology* (pp. 113-131). Washington, DC: American Psychiatric Press.

Riessman, C. K. (1993). *Narrative analysis: Qualitative research methods* (Vol. 30). Newbury Park, CA: Sage.

Russell, D. E. H. (1986). *The secret trauma: Incest in the lives of girls and women.* New York: Basic Books.

Schetky, D. H. (1990). A review of the literature on the long term effects of childhood sexual abuse. In R. P. Kluft (Ed.), *Incest-related syndromes of adult psychopathology* (pp. 35-44). Washington, DC: American Psychiatric Press.

Stevens, P. E., & Hall, J. M. (1991). A critical historical analysis of the medical construction of lesbianism. *International Journal of Health Services, 21*(2), 291-307.

Stivers, C. (1993). Reflections on the role of personal narrative in social science. *Signs: Journal of Women in Culture and Society, 18*(2), 408-425.

Stone, A. R. (1996). *The war of desire and technology at the close of the mechanical age.* Cambridge, MA: MIT Press.

U.S. Department of Labor. (1994). *Average annual pay levels in metropolitan areas, 1993.* Washington, DC: Bureau of Labor Statistics.

van der Kolk, B. A., McFarlane, A. C., & Weisaeth, L. (Eds.). (1996). *Traumatic stress: The effects of overwhelming experience on mind, body, and society.* New York: Guilford Press.

Domestic Violence in Lesbian Relationships: Findings of the Lesbian Relationships Research Project

Teresa Scherzer

SUMMARY. This article reports on the findings of the Lesbian Relationships Research Project (LRRP), a 1993 study on the prevalence of emotional and physical abuse in lesbian relationships in the San

---

Teresa Scherzer holds a Master of Social Work degree from San Francisco State University. To complete the MSW program, she and another MSW student conducted the Lesbian Relationships Research Project, and presented the study's findings at the National Lesbian and Gay Health Association annual conference in 1993. Ms. Scherzer has been a community activist and social worker in the San Francisco Bay Area for over 15 years, and has been a volunteer counselor and Board of Directors member for a local domestic violence agency. Currently she is a doctoral student in the medical sociology program at University of California San Francisco.

Address correspondence to: Teresa Scherzer, Department of Social and Behavioral Sciences, Box 0612, 521 Parnassus Avenue, University of California San Francisco, San Francisco, CA 94143.

The author wishes to acknowledge the invaluable collaboration with Christiane J. Medina, MSW, in conducting LRRP. The author also wishes to acknowledge the mentorship of Dr. Margo Okazawa-Rey and Dr. David O. Shipp, School of Social Work, San Francisco State University, and Dr. Howard Pinderhughes, Department of Social and Behavioral Sciences, UCSF.

[Haworth co-indexing entry note]: "Domestic Violence in Lesbian Relationships: Findings of the Lesbian Relationships Research Project." Scherzer, Teresa. Co-published simultaneously in *Journal of Lesbian Studies* (The Haworth Press, Inc.) Vol. 2, No. 1, 1998, pp. 29-47; and: *Gateways to Improving Lesbian Health and Health Care: Opening Doors* (ed: Christy M. Ponticelli) The Haworth Press, Inc., 1998, pp. 29-47; and: *Gateways to Improving Lesbian Health and Health Care: Opening Doors* (ed: Christy M. Ponticelli) Harrington Park Press, an imprint of The Haworth Press, Inc., 1998, pp. 29-47. Single or multiple copies of this article are available for a fee from The Haworth Document Delivery Service [1-800-342-9678, 9:00 a.m. - 5:00 p.m. (EST). E-mail address: getinfo@haworth.com].

Francisco Bay Area (Medina & Scherzer, 1993). This article reviews the literature on prevalence of domestic violence in lesbian relationships, describes the LRRP study, reports the findings from (1) the survey component of LRRP, which examined prevalence of specific abusive behaviors and respondents' help-seeking experiences, and (2) the qualitative component of the study, which asked respondents what behaviors they considered abusive, what happened when they sought help, and invited other comments. Lastly, the concepts and themes brought up from the qualitative data are discussed to suggest topics for further research. *[Article copies available for a fee from The Haworth Document Delivery Service: 1-800-342-9678. E-mail address: getinfo@haworth.com]*

INTRODUCTION

Domestic violence in lesbian relationships exists with the same violence, secrecy, and fear as in heterosexual battering relationships (Brand & Kidd, 1986; Hammond, 1989; Hart, 1986a; Kanuha, 1990; Kelly & Warshafsky, 1987; Leeder, 1988; Lobel, 1986; Renzetti, 1992). Although there appears to be increasing awareness of this issue within lesbian communities, there still exists a pervasive unwillingness of many lesbians to recognize domestic violence when it occurs, much less as an important issue in their communities. This article reports on the findings of the Lesbian Relationships Research Project (LRRP), a 1993 study on the reported frequency of abusive and violent behaviors in a sample of lesbian relationships in the San Francisco Bay Area (Medina & Scherzer, 1993). The 1993 study emphasized the frequency of reports of emotional and psychological abuse, and explored respondents' help-seeking experiences.

Often lesbian domestic violence is framed as "mutual" aggression and in general, it is taken less seriously than if the perpetrator were a man. The dominant culture's homophobia, racism, and sexism and the residual denial of same-sex domestic violence by other lesbians further exacerbates the secrecy, fear, and shame of lesbian victims and perpetrators. The relative invisibility of the issue and pervasive homophobia result in minimal support for lesbian victims of domestic violence within and outside lesbian communities. In the San Francisco Bay Area, however, many domestic violence agencies have implemented outreach and services specifically aimed at lesbian victims of domestic violence. Articles in community media, advertisements for services by different organizations, and other public discussion of this issue have helped to bring lesbian domestic violence more and more out of the closet.

In this article I explore lesbian domestic violence in its own right, and will not compare it to heterosexual domestic violence, although I do mention certain theoretical issues when relevant to the discussion. I do not explore the concept of "mutual aggression" except as this topic appears in the literature and as it pertains to implications for intervention.

In this article I review the literature on prevalence of domestic violence in lesbian relationships, describe the LRRP study, report the findings from (1) the survey component of LRRP, which examined reported frequencies of specific abusive behaviors and respondents' help-seeking experiences, and (2) the qualitative component of the study, which asked respondents what behaviors they considered abusive, what happened when they sought help, and invited other comments. Lastly, I address the concepts and themes that I interpreted from the qualitative data, in order to suggest topics for further research.

REVIEW OF THE LITERATURE

Five studies specifically examine the frequency of reported aggression in same-sex relationships (Bologna, Waterman, & Dawson, 1987, cited in Lie, Schilit, Bush, Montagne & Reyes, 1991; Brand & Kidd, 1986; Kelly & Warshafsky, 1987; Lie & Gentlewarrior, 1991; Lie et al., 1991). Popular estimates of the prevalence of same-sex domestic violence are based on these studies; however, none of these studies used random samples, which means, ultimately, that "prevalence" of aggression in same-sex relationships cannot be determined. We can only review the frequency of reported aggression in the study samples. This caveat is not to minimize the extent of same-sex domestic violence nor to trivialize these studies–it is simply to clarify its findings in light of the methodology.

The reported frequency of physically "aggressive" behavior in lesbian couples ranged from 25% (Brand & Kidd, 1986), to 40% being victimized and 54% using violence (Bologna et al., 1987, cited in Lie et al., 1991). Lie and Gentlewarrior (1991) found that 50.2% of their sample reported being victims, and that half of these women also used aggression toward their lovers. In a study of lesbians in currently "aggressive" relationships (Lie et al., 1991), 73.4% of respondents reported that in at least one previous lesbian relationship they had experienced some type of aggressive act.

Bologna et al. (1987) and Lie and Gentlewarrior (1991) found that subjects who reported using violence in a relationship also reported being victims of violence in that same relationship. For lesbians, those who used violence in current relationships also reported using violence in past relationships. "Reasons" for, or description of, the violence were not explored by either study. Moreover, all five research studies, and Renzetti's (1989, 1992) study, found that emotional, verbal, and psychological aggression were the most frequently reported, both in current and past relationships.

In an attempt to explore the use of aggression, Lie et al. (1991) concluded that the use of aggression in lesbian relationships may be viewed as "mutual aggression" or "a combination of self-defense and mutual aggression" (p. 134). Their conclusion suggests that aggression in lesbian relationships may not be based in a dynamic of domination and control, since the concept of two partners "mutually" using aggression against each other effectively shifts the focus of aggression away from any kind of power dynamic. Aggression is a tactic used to dominate another person. Self-defense speaks to an individual using physical force to protect herself from aggression. "Mutual aggression" serves theoretically to remove the dynamic of control from the relationship in which "aggression" is reported.

The conclusions of Lie et al. (1991) directly conflict with nearly all of the lesbian and general domestic violence literature–the personal testimony of survivors of lesbian abuse, professional case studies on lesbian domestic violence, and writers and activists/advocates for battered lesbians (Hammond, 1989; Hart, 1986a, 1986b; Leeder, 1988; Renzetti, 1989, 1992). Hart (1986a) succinctly stated:

> Lesbian battering is that pattern of violent and coercive behaviors whereby a lesbian seeks to control the thoughts, beliefs or conduct of her intimate partner or to punish the intimate for resisting the perpetrator's control over her. Individual acts of physical violence, by this definition, do not constitute lesbian battering. Physical violence is not battering unless it results in the enhanced control of the batterer over the recipient. (p. 173)

The literature discusses the manipulation and confusion concerning accountability for domestic violence. Domestic violence victims will often blame themselves for the abuse (Hart, 1986a; Walker, 1979; Walker, 1986) and batterers will often reinforce this belief to further control the victim and avoid accountability. Lesbian victims may fight back more than heterosexual women (Porat, 1986; Walker, 1986), and their aggression may cause them to blame themselves even more for the abuse inflicted upon them. Perpetrators often feel they are the victims, especially if both women in the couple use physical or verbal aggression (Hammond, 1989), or when the victim withdraws after an abusive incident (Walker, 1986).

Similarities to and differences from heterosexual domestic violence have been explored by many researchers (Brand & Kidd, 1986; Hart, 1986a; Kanuha, 1990; Renzetti, 1989, 1992). Renzetti (1989, 1992) offers insight into the dynamics and correlates of abuse in lesbian relationships. Many definitive characteristics of heterosexual domestic violence are clearly present in abusive lesbian relationships (Hammond, 1989; Leeder, 1988; Lobel, 1986) such as the phenomenon Walker (1979) defined as the "battering cycle" or the cycle of violence. Other characteristics of domestic violence include: perpetrators' tactics of isolation and breaking down victims' self-esteem, the self-blame of the victims who assume responsibility for the abuse and violence, and perpetrators' patterns of control using manipulative, intimidating, or violent behavior.

Unique to lesbian relationships are the chronic and cumulative effects of a homophobic world that imposes tremendous stress on the process of developing a healthy sense of self and healthy relationships with others (Hammond, 1989; Leeder, 1988; Lobel, 1986). The lack of social validation and open hostility lead many lesbians, as well as other members of oppressed groups, to be insular and protective of each other and their relationships (Krestan & Bepko, 1980, cited in Renzetti, 1992; Lobel, 1986). Individuals and communities deny or minimize the extent that lesbians are abusive or violent to their lovers. This denial is especially painful when a battered lesbian approaches friends for help, who then deny the reality of the situation. Moreover, the insensitivity or hostility of mainstream institutions prevents lesbians from seeking or receiving help from police or from helping professionals (Hammond, 1989; Leeder, 1988; Lobel, 1986).

In sum, the literature on domestic violence between lesbian intimates is a body of work that includes the personal testimony of survivors, and professional articles and research studies by clinicians and academicians. There is a definite clarity and consistency among the personal accounts on the elements and dynamics of lesbian battering. Recent research by Renzetti (1989, 1992) helps document that lesbian domestic violence is a serious issue, and explores correlates of abuse, such as dependency and autonomy, jealousy, and substance abuse. Renzetti's research is extremely valuable, since by exploring victims' experiences, she offers significant insight into the complexity of domestic violence in lesbian relationships. In particular, Renzetti explored victims' help-seeking experiences and let their voices tell readers what responses were or would have been most helpful.

A gap in the literature is the lack of empirical data on psychological or emotional abuse. The absence or omission of research on this kind of abuse reinforces its "invisibility" as "abuse," the belief that it is not as severe or as damaging to the victim as physical abuse. Many researchers have written that the participants in their studies stated that the psychological abuse was more frequent and equally or more destructive than any physical abuse (Brand & Kidd, 1986; Renzetti, 1989, 1992; Walker, 1979).

Another significant gap in the literature concerns the low priority assigned to the voices and experiences of lesbians of color. At best, samples included 13% women of color (Lie & Gentlewarrior, 1991). This rather monochromatic picture of lesbians, as with the lack of data on emotional abuse, served to reinforce invisibility and marginalization of many lesbians. Invisibility and an ensuing lack of appropriate services continue to negatively impact significant segments of the lesbian population.

METHODOLOGY

Research Design

The purpose of the Lesbian Relationships Research Project (Medina & Scherzer, 1993) was three-fold:

1. to gather information regarding the reported frequency of abusive or violent behaviors in a sample of lesbian relationships in the San Francisco Bay Area,
2. to assess respondents' attitudes and beliefs about abusive or violent behaviors,
3. to review respondents' help-seeking experiences.

Another major purpose of LRRP was to validate the experiences of survivors of lesbian domestic violence. As the original report stated:

> For these women, it may finally give name to this very insidious type of abuse which so often goes unchecked, and can lead to devastating consequences including the decimation of their self-esteem. The final purpose of the project, then, was for the questionnaire to serve as a mode of intervention, as a consciousness-raising tool for participants to question "what is abuse?" about their own and others' situations. (Medina & Scherzer, 1993, pp. 3-4)

LRRP was a descriptive, cross-sectional study that utilized an anonymous, self-administered questionnaire. Women who self-identified as lesbians were asked to report on their demographics, on behaviors that occurred in their current or most recent lesbian relationship, and on their attitudes and beliefs regarding domestic violence.

Potential indicators and examples of emotional and physical abuse, as well as behaviors associated with domestic violence, were identified from the domestic violence literature (Hart, 1986a, 1986b; Renzetti, 1989, 1992; Walker, 1979; White, 1985; Zambrano, 1985) and were operationalized. The behaviors selected were those most frequently mentioned in personal testimonies of victims of lesbian domestic violence in the works of Lobel (1986) and Renzetti (1989, 1992) as present in most or all battering relationships. The questionnaire included two open-ended questions about help-seeking experiences and what other behaviors respondents thought were abusive, and in a third "open space" invited respondents to make any comments. To address a bias of social desirability (Rubin & Babbie, 1989), and to address the shifting of blame that frequently occurs in abusive relationships, Medina and Scherzer (1993) structured questions to appear nonjudgmental, and included the two open-ended questions for respondents to tell their stories in their own words.

Variables

The variables in the study included demographic variables such as age, race/ethnicity, education level, income, role identification (butch or femme), degree of being "out" as a lesbian, relationship status (single or partnered), motherhood, and disability. Other variables were: frequency of emotional abuse, frequency of physical abuse, "comfort" with disagreements or fights, ability to ask for help, use of helping resources, and perceptions of abuse (which included attitudes and beliefs about a range of behaviors, and other behaviors respondents could describe in the open-ended questions).

Instrument

The instrument was a six-page, 88-item, anonymous, self-administered questionnaire that was ready to be mailed after the respondent finished. A detachable informed consent cover sheet provided information about who the researchers were, the study's purpose, the name and phone number of the faculty supervisor, and a statement assuring the respondent's anonymity. In addition, a partial listing of lesbian-sensitive domestic violence and mental health resources was included for respondents, in the event that their participation in the study raised issues they wished to talk about.

The questionnaire covered five areas of concern. The first section asked respondents about their demographic characteristics. The following two sections addressed "Disagreement and Compromise" in relationships. Here, respondents were asked to report on the frequency of their own behaviors, and on their partners' behaviors, which operationalized "power over" and "control." The next section was a modified Conflict Tactics Scale (Straus, 1979) that served as a global indicator of abuse in the relationship. Medina and Scherzer (1993) modified the Conflict Tactics Scale to emphasize emotional abuse, and to include behaviors having particular resonance for lesbians (e.g., threats to "out" a partner). Following this was a series of questions about how respondents viewed fights or disagreements, and about their help-seeking experiences, if any. The final section questioned respondents' general attitudes and beliefs regarding what constitutes abusive behavior in a relationship.

LRRP's measure of abuse was based on Straus's Conflict Tactics Scale (1979) and included two behavior clusters of emotional and physical abuse. Victimization by emotional abuse was indicated by a positive response to questions of being verbally put down in front of friends or relatives, insulting or swearing at lover, threatening to commit suicide, and other similar behaviors. In this section, respondents were asked if during a disagreement or fight had *either* they or their partners ever engaged in any of the behaviors. By structuring questions this way, Medina and Scherzer hoped to minimize under-reporting, and elicit more truthful reporting.

To examine respondents' help-seeking experiences, the instrument included a checklist and an open-ended question that respondents were to complete only if they viewed the way disagreements and/or fights were handled in their relationship as a problem. This section asked respondents whether they felt able to ask for help; if not, what prevented them; if yes, where did they go, and what happened when they sought help.

In light of the dynamics where perpetrators often feel they are the victims, and where victims may assume responsibility for the abuse, respondents were not asked whether they identified as a victim or as a perpetrator; instead, Medina and Scherzer wanted to see how they described the situation using their own words. Respondents' comments, as well as their forced-choice responses in "Disagreement and Compromise" often suggested power and abuse issues in the relationship, beyond the basic reporting of certain behaviors.

Outreach and Data Collection

Data collection methods utilized both snowball sampling and having the surveys available in public places. Nonrandom sampling methods were selected in order to ensure a racially diverse sample, despite the fact that, as in previous studies (Bologna et al., 1987, cited in Lie et al., 1991; Brand & Kidd, 1986; Kelly & Warshafsky, 1987; Lie & Gentlewarrior, 1991; Lie et al., 1991), findings from nonrandom samples cannot be used to generalize to a larger population. Medina and Scherzer contacted women in their various professional and personal networks asking for their help in distributing the survey. The researchers also contacted businesses, organizations, and agencies that serve lesbians, and asked them, when possible, to advertise the research project and make the questionnaire available to any interested lesbian. In addition, Medina and Scherzer contacted Bay Area domestic violence agencies to inform them of the project and to invite the participation of staff and clients. By engaging key members of different lesbian communities of color, of old/er lesbians, of young/er lesbians, members of important community resources, the questionnaire was distributed to a broad range of communities.

An information packet was prepared that included a general cover letter and a copy of the questionnaire, with a copy of the Human Subjects Protocol approval, to send to key prospects in the outreach. In order to personalize the project and enhance community links and participation, a personalized cover letter introduced the researchers and the project.

RESULTS

Description of the Sample

Of the approximately 650 questionnaires distributed to individuals and made available in public places, 258 were returned. A total of 256 usable surveys, surpassing the goal of 200, constituted the final sample.

Nearly half of the respondents (47%) were between the ages of 31 and 40 years old, with 29% between 21 and 30, and 20% between 41 and 50. The sample's level of education was high, with over 97% of respondents reporting at least some college education. Forty-four percent were college graduates, and 32% had advanced degrees. Income levels were somewhat evenly distributed, with the largest number of respondents (31%) reporting $20,000-29,999.

The racial diversity of the sample is a result of the intensive outreach and community participation. Nearly half the sample (44%) were women of color. Asian and Pacific Islander women constituted 12%, Native women constituted 2%, women of African descent constituted 10%, Latinas constituted 10%, and women who are multiracial, Arab, or who identified in other ways constituted 11% (figure exceeds 100% due to rounding).

Role identification was not a major issue for 71% of respondents, who did not identify with roles, or who identified with both/either; and the remaining 29% of respondents were evenly divided between "mostly butch" and "mostly femme." The degree to which respondents were "out" was generally high, with 58% reporting that 100% of the people in their life knew they were lesbians, and 29% of the sample reporting 75%. Eighty percent of respondents reported being in a current relationship, and 14% had children. Fourteen percent of respondents reported a disability, with the vast majority reporting Chronic Fatigue Immune Dysfunction Syndrome or Environmental Illness.

Reported Frequency of Emotional or Physical Abuse

Seventeen (17%) percent of respondents reported experiencing physical abuse at some time during their current or most recent relationship, and 31% reported experiencing emotional abuse. The specific frequency distributions are illustrated in Tables 1 and 2.

The question of frequency was further enhanced by respondents' com-

TABLE 1. Reported Frequency of Physical Abuse (N = 256)

	n =	%
Pushed, grabbed, or shoved the other	63	25%
Slapped, kicked, bit or hit the other	38	15%
Forced public displays of sexual behavior	10	4%
Drove recklessly to punish or scare the other	62	24%
Disrupted or impeded the other's eating or sleeping habits	80	31%
Abused the other's children or own	5	14%*

**of 37 respondents who had children; 2% of entire sample*

TABLE 2. Reported Frequency of Emotional Abuse (N = 256)

	n =	%
Insulted or swore at the other	171	67%
Threw, smashed, hit or kicked something	116	45%
Threatened to expose the other as a lesbian	7	3%
Verbally put down the other in front of strangers	57	22%
Verbally put down the other in front of friends/relatives	83	32%
Threatened to commit suicide	35	14%

ments in the open-ended questions and comments sections. Thirteen respondents wrote that, although their current relationships were not abusive or violent, their previous ones were. Three other respondents wrote that major changes had occurred in their long-term relationships, where abuse had occurred earlier, but had stopped. Another respondent wrote that although she herself had not experienced an abusive relationship, numerous lesbian friends had been physically and sexually abused by their partners, many of them recently.

Help-Seeking Experiences

Over half the sample, 137 participants (53.5%), reported viewing fights or disagreements as problems. As shown in Table 3, of these 137 women, 115 reported asking for help. Of these 115 respondents, 54 reported going to one helping resource, 45 went to two resources, and 26 respondents went to three or more resources.

Other types of help sought by respondents included "talking it out," "mediation," twelve-step groups or sponsors, support from coworkers/supervisor. Couples counseling was a helping resource that numerous respondents wrote in the "Other help" fill-in section, although it was coded as "Counseling."

Chi square analyses revealed no significant differences between "Race" and ability to ask for help ($\chi^2 = 7.016$, df = 10, p = .72). No

TABLE 3. Where Did Respondents Seek Help? (n = 115)

	n =
Counselor	90
Friend	82
Parent	9
Other Family	18
Police	6
Domestic Violence Agency	5
Doctor	2
Crisis Line	4
Religious Counselor	3
Legal Assistance	3
Other Help	16

significant differences were found between "Race" and the two most utilized helping resources, Counselor ($\chi^2 = 7.846$, df = 10, p = .64) and Friend ($\chi^2 = 6.603$, df = 10, p = .76).

Sixty-four respondents (25%) reported that they felt unable to seek help for several reasons (see Table 4). Forty women cited one reason, 13 cited two reasons, and 11 respondents cited three or more reasons. Some respondents who utilized helping resources also reported feeling unable to seek help at other times for different reasons.

The "other reasons" cited by respondents in the fill-in section included a fear of breaking up with partner, feelings of guilt, feeling "crazy," and feeling that the problems were their fault.

Qualitative Data Analysis

The results from the forced-choice responses do not tell us about the perceptions and experiences of the respondents, nor the impact that abusive acts have on the individual to whom they are directed. For this reason the LRRP questionnaire (Medina & Scherzer, 1993) included open-ended questions and room for comments, so respondents could share their experiences and perceptions in their own words.

"What happened when you sought help?"

Responses to this open-ended question, and respondents' other comments often suggested whether or not a relationship was abusive, or if problems were due to communication difficulties or other non-abusive themes. Twenty-seven respondents wrote that they learned better communication skills, that "things worked out," that they learned to set better boundaries, and other similar responses. However, 15 women who wrote

TABLE 4. What Prevented Respondents from Seeking Help? (n = 64)

	n =
Embarrassment	14
Money	15
Fear of retaliation	5
Didn't know where to seek help	7
Fear of insensitivity to lesbians	9
Other reasons	17

apparently benign comments about boundaries later revealed that they or their partners were emotionally or physically abusive.

Seven respondents wrote that "help" did not work out because the partner would not participate in some way to work together through the issues. One respondent wrote "Still didn't seem resolved–my partner was unable or unwilling to follow through on the compromises agreed to–situation remained back to the same."

Counseling, although the most heavily utilized resource, sometimes appeared to threaten respondents and their partners. One woman wrote she and her partner went to couples counseling, after seeking individual or group counseling through a domestic violence agency; the respondent wrote that she felt "guilty" because the agency staff portrayed the partner as "worse than she is." Another respondent reported that she and her partner went to couples and individual counseling, but her partner felt threatened and "feared therapist would turn [respondent] against her." A third woman said that she did not want to go to counseling because she feared discovering she and her partner were "incompatible." Still another woman wrote that she had seen "helpers" but did not like how "Lesbian Feminist Therapists" [*sic*] seem to be instrumental in splitting up other couples.

Two respondents reported that helping resources were themselves actual barriers to service. One respondent wrote that she and her partner were denied service by a lesbian agency: "I told a lesbian mental health center we were s/m dykes and was informed we could not get help. They did not deal with 'us.'" Another respondent wrote that the lesbian domestic violence program she sought help from was "disorganized" and "inefficient"; she went to another agency, which assisted her with a restraining order and court accompaniment. A third woman wrote of her fear that the agency she went to would be insensitive to lesbians.

The comments of eight respondents who sought and received help from different sources seemed to suggest that they were the partners who were abusive. Nearly all respondents who disclosed acting abusively "explained" why, often citing childhood abuse or other victimization, personal or institutional. One woman wrote she sought help from friends, domestic violence agencies, counseling, and 12-step groups: "Helped create boundaries and tools for coping. Facilitated better communication." However, her later comments said "Many of us in abusive relationships are ACAs [Adult Children of Alcoholics], incest survivors, eco. [economically] disadvantaged . . . all contributing to . . . hitting out violently or abusively."

Another respondent who wrote that she went to friends and other family members, and "got support and reassurance that I was not necessarily at fault" also wrote "Important to note fear as well as anger. One can be manipulated by fear which can lead to abusive behavior." Another respondent wrote that "friends listened and gave advice"; she also wrote that she was sexually abused as a child, and as an adult, physically abused intimate others when she was "under the influence of alcohol or drugs."

Respondents who revealed they were victims, however, did not offer "reasons" for their behavior. Eleven women, answering "What happened when you sought help?" wrote "Not much," "nothing," or "temporary relief." They described feeling "crazy," protective of their partner, internalizing blame. One respondent wrote, "I felt that the violence toward me was my fault even if I knew better." Another wrote that she felt "guilty" because her situation "was not serious enough." Still another wrote, "when she used violence against me, I wanted to turn her in but I just couldn't because I felt like no one could help her feel better but herself and me . . . if she were a man I would have had her arrested for battery for sure . . . "

One respondent who reported much violence ("Often" and "Always" categories in the Conflict Tactics/Abuse section) wrote: "My partner has said [that] if I see someone I will be committed. She says I'm crazy and its [*sic*] my problem." She also wrote "scary shit to think about . . . good to have the phone numbers."

What other behaviors did respondents consider abusive?

Respondents' perceptions of what constitutes abusive behavior were often revealed in their comments about what other behaviors they considered abusive. Many respondents considered other abusive behaviors to include: threatening to "out" the other, "racist comments," theft of money and valuables, "drama," "push-pull behavior," "emotional and mental manipulation," "economic control, holding children in the relationship hostage," leaving harassing messages (written and on answering machine), property destruction, insulting respondent's friends and family members, and not allowing respondent to have time alone. The domestic violence literature consistently agrees that these behaviors are abusive.

Six respondents considered other abusive behaviors to be: "shared private info with others," and "talking to friends about couple's relationship problems." Nowhere in the literature are these behaviors considered abusive towards another person. The comments may reflect power and control issues of the respondents, by suggesting a strong focus on privacy that might be construed as the respondents' attempts to monitor or control the partners who are talking to other people. The comments may suggest the dynamics that Cecere (1986) described when she wrote "I allowed [the batterer] to convince me that I was the one who instigated the abuse. It seems that anytime my needs differed from hers, I was being abusive" (p. 26). However, the comments may also reflect a difference in cultural attitudes and beliefs. Given the diversity among lesbians, it is difficult, if not dangerous, to generalize; cultural contexts should be examined before any conclusions are drawn.

LIMITATIONS OF THE STUDY

The questionnaire yielded informative data of the reported frequency of both psychological and physical abuse that served to demonstrate that physical or emotional abuse was not an anomalous report in the sample. The survey instrument, however, although constructed using the experiences of survivors of lesbian domestic violence, was not tested for validity and reliability. In addition, the frequencies of reported aggression reported in the quantitative part of the survey viewed in light of the attitudes, beliefs, and perceptions revealed by respondents in the qualitative part strongly suggest that a quantitative analysis of a relationship's power dynamics, beyond the basic reporting of abusive behaviors, would be much less fruitful than a future study utilizing qualitative methods. Qualitative methods could capture "power dynamics" as it exists as a processual and dynamic relationship between two individuals.

The study's findings are limited by the nonrandom sampling methods and thus cannot be generalized beyond the sample to a larger population. Due to the sampling methods, there are no data to compare respondents with women who did not participate in the study. Moreover, the findings are based on the reports of abuse by the respondents, and actual prevalence of lesbian domestic violence may be different than what was reported in the study. Domestic violence is a very under-reported crime (Walker, 1979), and many women who are currently in abusive relationships may not have the psychological or physical freedom to participate in a survey. This survey asked respondents to report only on their current or most recent relationships, and several respondents wrote that if they had been asked about earlier relationships, their answers would have been very different. Prevalence is also difficult to assess due to batterers' unwillingness to participate in domestic violence research (Walker, 1979); and, if they do, may minimize or deny their abusive behavior (Hart, 1986b; Walker, 1979).

DISCUSSION

The LRRP found that emotional and physical abuse in San Francisco Bay Area lesbian relationships was reported in approximately one out of three, and one out of six relationships, respectively. That emotional abuse was reported more frequently than physical abuse is consistent with the literature (Brand & Kidd, 1986; Renzetti, 1989, 1992; Walker, 1979). Higher reporting of victim-behaviors than perpetrator-behaviors may reflect a bias of social desirability (Rubin & Babbie, 1989). Also consistent with the literature is the perception of many perpetrators to offer "reasons" for their abusive or violent behavior, and the perception of many victims to feel at fault for the abuse (Hammond, 1989; Hart, 1986a; Renzetti, 1989, 1992; Walker, 1979).

Forty-four percent of the respondents were women of color, and the study's findings show that there was no significant difference among any of the racial groups and the reporting of abusive behaviors, which contradicts the suggestion that violence may be "more rare in minority lesbian relationships" (Renzetti, 1992, p. 14). The findings further tell us that no differences were revealed between racial groups in feeling able to ask for help, and seeking help from different resources.

Most respondents sought to reconcile relationship problems on their own, with friends, with individual counselors, or through couples counseling. Some respondents describe problems of communication; some directly speak of emotional or physical abuse. Only nine out of the 115 women who sought help (8%) approached domestic violence agencies and called crisis lines. Interestingly, despite the large numbers of lesbian services in the San Francisco Bay Area, numerous women wrote that they did not know where to go for help. Unfortunately there are no data to explore this issue further.

The questionnaire's role as a thought-provoking vehicle, for participants to re-evaluate their own and others' experiences, especially regarding underlying power dynamics that may exist in relationships, was a research objective that was successfully met. Medina and Scherzer (1993) received many comments by respondents about how they viewed and utilized the questionnaire as such a tool. As Medina and Scherzer (1993) had hoped, numerous questions were raised during the completion process, among them:

- What is abuse?
- If I see these behaviors, what does it mean? and what should I do?
- Do I hold a double standard regarding assessment of heterosexual versus lesbian domestic violence?

The LRRP succeeded in gathering a large sample that was much more racially diverse than in previous studies, but the nonrandom sampling method does not lend itself to generalizations of the population beyond the study sample. With the qualitative data from the respondents, however, we can learn much about the dynamics of lesbian domestic violence in the San Francisco Bay Area by the reports of the examples of psychological and physical abuse, respondents' perceptions about conflict and abuse, and help-seeking experiences of the respondents.

CONCLUSIONS

Implications for Intervention

Despite the relatively high degree of consciousness and sensitivity in the Bay Area towards lesbian domestic violence, lesbians in abusive relationships face numerous barriers to intervention and service. Often when battered lesbians call domestic violence agencies, many battered lesbians do not disclose their batterer's gender for fear of homophobic reaction by service providers or other clients. Lesbian batterers who do seek help face a lack of services even more scarce than those for victims, since most services for batterers are for men, and are greatly outnumbered by services for victims. Moreover, many lesbian batterers believe that they are the victims of their partners, and will seek (and receive) help as victims, by the lesbian domestic violence programs set up to serve the "real" victims of lesbian domestic violence.

An issue that is especially problematic in providing services and in recognizing and naming domestic violence is the difficulty of assessing who is the victim and who is the perpetrator. Many lesbian and gay, as well as heterosexual, service providers and criminal justice personnel, argue that same-sex domestic violence does not fit a heterosexual model, and is actually "mutual battering." Because the roles in same-sex relationships are far less clear than in heterosexual relationships, individuals and communities often project an attitude that same-sex domestic violence is not as serious nor as prevalent as domestic violence in heterosexual relationships, and the issue is often not addressed appropriately. This lack of understanding and appropriate interventions for victims and batterers means that the former do not receive help or protection, and that the latter are under practically no pressure to be accountable for their abusive and violent behavior. In light of respondents' preferred resource of counseling, the need for heightened sensitivity of mental health professionals regarding the complexity of lesbian domestic violence becomes increasingly urgent.

Future Research

The survey component of LRRP gathered information on the reported frequency of abusive behaviors, while the qualitative data indicates patterns of conflict and interaction that may suggest underlying power dynamics and domestic violence. Future research could collect data that could illuminate the psychological elements of these interactions, especially the underlying power dynamics.

One question that LRRP raised was whether domestic violence in lesbian relationships does genuinely involve shifting of power relations between the partners, or if shifts occur from relationship to relationship. In other words, if someone is battered in her current relationship, will she ever become a batterer herself, either in her current relationship or in a subsequent one? Another issue for future research to tackle is that of "mutual aggression"– does abuse or violence in lesbian relationships ever exist within a genuinely "mutual" pattern, where neither partner continually dominates the other? These questions must be answered through careful and conscientious social science research, where qualitative data may be gathered so that the women can tell their stories in their own voices. We then may be able to view a more three-dimensional picture of lesbian domestic violence, and may be able to answer the questions LRRP, and others, have raised.

REFERENCES

Brand, P.A., & Kidd, A. H. (1986). Frequency of physical aggression in heterosexual and female homosexual dyads. *Psychological Reports*, *59*, 1307-1313.

Cecere, D. J. (1986). The second closet: Battered lesbians. In K. Lobel (Ed.), *Naming the violence: Speaking out about lesbian battering* (pp. 21-31). Seattle: Seal Press.

Hammond, N. (1988). Lesbian victims of relationship violence. *Women and Therapy*, *8* (1-2), 89-105.

Hart, B. (1986a). Lesbian battering: An examination. In K. Lobel (Ed.), *Naming the violence: Speaking out about lesbian battering* (pp. 173-200). Seattle: Seal Press.

Hart, B. (1986b). Safe space for battered lesbians. In K. Lobel (Ed.), *Naming the violence: Speaking out about lesbian battering* (pp. 95-97). Seattle: Seal Press.

Kanuha, V. (1990). Compounding the triple jeopardy: Battering in lesbian of color relationships. *Women and Therapy*, *9* (1-2), 169-184.

Kelly, E.E., & Warshafsky, L. (1987, July). Partner abuse in gay male and lesbian couples. Paper presented at the Third National Conference for Family Violence Researchers, Durham, N.H.

Leeder, E. (1988). Enmeshed in pain: Counseling the lesbian battering couple. *Women and Therapy, 7* (1), 81-99.

Lie, G.-Y., & Gentlewarrior, S. (1991). Intimate violence in lesbian relationships: Discussion of survey findings and practice implications. *Journal of Social Service Research, 15* (1-2), 41-59.

Lie, G.-Y., Schilit, R., Bush, J., Montagne, M., & Reyes, L. (1991). Lesbians in currently aggressive relationships: How frequently do they report aggressive past relationships? *Violence and Victims, 6* (2), 121-135.

Lobel, K. (Ed.). (1986). *Naming the violence: Speaking out about lesbian battering*. Seattle: Seal Press.

Medina, C.J., & Scherzer, T. (1993). *The Lesbian Relationships Research Project.* Unpublished Master's of Social Work research project, San Francisco State University, San Francisco, CA.

Porat, N. (1986). Support groups for battered lesbians. In K. Lobel (Ed.), *Naming the violence: Speaking out about lesbian battering* (pp. 80-87). Seattle: Seal Press.

Renzetti, C. M. (1989). Building a second closet: Third party responses to victims of lesbian partner abuse. *Family Relations, 38*, 157-163.

Renzetti, C. M. (1992). *Violent betrayal: Partner abuse in lesbian relationships.* Newbury Park, CA: Sage.

Rubin, A., & Babbie, E. (1989). *Research methods for social work*. Belmont, CA: Wadsworth.

Straus, M. A. (1979). Measuring intrafamily conflict and violence: The conflict tactics (ct) scales. *Journal of Marriage and the Family, 41*, 75-88.

Walker, L. E. (1979). *The battered woman*. New York: Harper & Row.

Walker, L. (1986). Battered women's shelters and work with battered lesbians. In K. Lobel (Ed.), *Naming the violence: Speaking out about lesbian battering* (pp. 73-76). Seattle: Seal Press.

White, E. C. (1985). *Chain, chain, change: For black women dealing with physical and emotional abuse*. Seattle: Seal Press.

Zambrano, M. J. (1985). *Mejor sola que mal acompañada: Para la mujer golpeada/for the Latina in an abusive relationship*. Seattle: Seal Press.

Lesbian Pass/ages: Invisible Lives and Issues of Community

Barbara Isaac
Barbara M. Herringer

SUMMARY. Despite the greater inclusion of women in the recent literature on aging, lesbians continue to remain invisible. This article presents the inquiries of two mid-life lesbian social work academics into the lives of lesbian women growing older, and the gaps revealed between the images of lesbians constructed in the public domain, and the lives of women who do not fit the mainstream or dominant images. The inquiry begins with the voices of the "experts": women who are living their mid-life years as lesbians in a society which does not "see" or image them. Whether or not this invisibility in mid-life and old age can be overcome through access to a supportive community seems open to debate. *[Article copies available for a fee from The Haworth Document Delivery Service: 1-800-342-9678. E-mail address: getinfo@haworth.com]*

Barbara Isaac is Assistant Professor in the College of Arts, Social and Health Sciences/Social Work at University of Northern British Columbia, and holds a cross-appointment in Women's Studies/Gender Studies. Her research interests include women's health, working-class lives, and feminist pedagogy. Barbara M. Herringer is Associate Professor in the College of Arts, Social and Health Sciences/Social Work at University of Northern British Columbia and holds a cross-appointment in Women's Studies/Gender Studies. Among her research interests are HIV/AIDS suicide; the effects of child welfare policy on women; and lesbian health/culture.

Address correspondence to: Barbara Isaac, College of Arts, Social and Health Sciences/Social Work, University of Northern British Columbia, 3333 University Way, Prince George, BC V2N 4Z9, Canada.

[Haworth co-indexing entry note]: "Lesbian Pass/ages: Invisible Lives and Issues of Community." Isaac, Barbara, and Barbara M. Herringer. Co-published simultaneously in *Journal of Lesbian Studies* (The Haworth Press, Inc.) Vol. 2, No. 1, 1998, pp. 49-59; and: *Gateways to Improving Lesbian Health and Health Care: Opening Doors* (ed: Christy M. Ponticelli) The Haworth Press, Inc., 1998, pp. 49-59; and: *Gateways to Improving Lesbian Health and Health Care: Opening Doors* (ed: Christy M. Ponticelli) Harrington Park Press, an imprint of The Haworth Press, Inc., 1998, pp. 49-59. Single or multiple copies of this article are available for a fee from The Haworth Document Delivery Service [1-800-342-9678, 9:00 a.m. - 5:00 p.m. (EST). E-mail address: getinfo@haworth.com].

> Years ago when I was walking downtown, I was just in the process of coming out, and I saw an older woman who looked disenfranchised. She was probably about the age I am now. And I thought, the moment I say I'm a lesbian that's what's going to happen to me. I'm going to be old, lonely and have nowhere to live. That was my greatest fear. Then I came out as a lesbian and that didn't happen at all.
>
> Now that feeling is coming back–not because I'm a lesbian, but because I'm realizing that there were all those years I was not ageless. I knew I was growing older but I didn't want to grow old. But now I'm realizing not only am I growing older, I'm getting old. And I'm aware of what that means–the possibility of being alone, being poor, of not having control over my life, over what I do and where I live. And I think, I'm under the grand illusion that if I was heterosexual and with a man these thoughts wouldn't be occurring to me . . . because I'd be too busy taking care of other people.

As over-40 lesbian social work academics concerned with women's social and health issues we recently hosted a dinner especially to bring lesbians "of a certain age" together to talk about images of aging, the processes of aging, the invisibility of aging lesbians in cultural, health and policy contexts, and lesbian social issues in general. Our interests in the lives of women growing older emerged not only from our own experiences, but also from social work studies exploring the thoughts and experiences of contemporary spinsters both lesbian and heterosexual (Isaac & Herringer, 1996; Gallagher, 1996; Herringer, 1991). Our inquiries revealed significant gaps between the images of women constructed in the public domain, and the lives of women who do not fit the mainstream or dominant images. As lesbians who are among those not present in the public eye, we chose to begin our work with the voices of the "experts"–women who are living their mid-life years as lesbians in a society which does not "see" or image them.

When we discover our *self* in relation to another woman it transforms the landscape and the communities to which we belong. Speaking or writing as lesbians about our everyday lives, unmasks what others call the forbidden. It explodes the language we grew up with–transforms it into mother tongue. Mother tongue is a familiar but dangerous site when we begin speaking out in the world. As one woman told others at dinner:

> I'm always tempted, when I help someone out in a tight situation, to say "well, you've just been helped by a lesbian."

Being "tempted" brings into relief that we do not yet have our "tongues," our voices, our full lives. Imaging, imagining, eyeing, making eye contact.

Images of aging until recently conjured a generic or universal old person. Slowly, with the urging of feminist practitioners and academics (often those of us moving into middle age) as well as older women themselves, public images of aging women began to appear. It seemed so obvious. Older women were the majority in our culture; yet we knew little about them, and saw even less in media images. Elderly women when portrayed at all, were pictured as mirror images or reflections of the men with whom they lived, or had lived–usually white, middle-class, heterosexual, often educated. The images were often constructed according to their caring roles in relation to children/grandchildren, and yet in many instances, their lives and experiences were assumed to be the same as men. While recent gerontological research has succeeded in claiming some space for older women (Neugarten, 1982; Gee & Kimball, 1987), images of those who remained single has continued to be sparse. While there is little information on spinsters (Herringer, 1991; Jeffreys, 1985; Simon, 1987), there is less about older lesbians, or as some prefer to name themselves–dykes or queers (Gallagher, 1996). If older "dominant" or mainstream women are barely visible, then these "other" old women are hidden beneath even thicker shrouds. Furthermore, any public recognition of the word lesbian attaches itself to a particular history that ignores women of colour, aboriginal women and class. If positive images exist, it is difficult to find them. What does exist tells us that lesbians may be married, single, divorced, mothers, from all classes, all occupations, races and cultures, religions, disabled or able-bodied, different shapes and sizes. As Auger (1990) notes: "Lesbians who are old are . . . in triple jeopardy . . . They are not young, they do not enjoy the privilege of patriarchal masculinity, and they do not receive the social rewards of heterosexuality. Those who are not white suffer yet another stigma, as do those who are differently abled [or poor]" (p. 26).

Responses to the needs of women in Canada reflect the influence and power of society and its institutions (Bishop, 1994; Mullaly, 1993). Women, particularly working class, lesbian and visible minorities, continue to be marginalized; consequently, little real work has been undertaken to address needs applicable to the wide variation of our lives. Indeed, most cultural and political structures aimed at women have been designed explicitly to portray them or benefit them in their capacity as wives and mothers. As a result, women as individual subjects continue to be obscured and are regarded primarily in relation to others. Even in this context, however, only certain relations are recognized. No single experience speaks for all; yet where are any of our experiences and lives reflected/imaged? As with the word spinster that conjures an ugly and passionless old woman (Hufton, 1984; Jeffreys, 1985; Vicinus, 1985), most concepts of lesbian evoke images of non-women who look and act like men, or who hate both children and men. Whether as spinsters and/or as lesbians we are perceived as a threat to the social order. It is deviancy that others imagine when women, either through choice or circumstance do not marry and have children, or whose primary relationships are with women. One of our dinner/discussion participants remarked that in her experience,

> People look for visible clues, they say, 'if they're not visible to me . . . if I wouldn't recognize them on the street, then they don't exist.' They wouldn't know a lesbian if they tripped over one because they're looking for something different. We're dealing with differences that are invisible. We're trying to make ourselves visible. It's hard to be out there and recognize what we need for ourselves.

Ideas and images about aging and of lesbianism continue to rely on assumptions of who women *should* be (Herringer, 1991; Isaac & Herringer, 1996). Despite feminist inroads, policy and research concerning women in mid-life are often based on the assumption that all women in this age group are, or were, married and have children, and are heterosexual (Gee & Kimball, 1987; McCannell, McCarthy & Herringer, 1990; McCannell & Herringer, 1992; Giele, 1982; Zones, Estes & Binney, 1987). Until recently, the common shared experience (and image) of women between 40 and 60 was that of homemaker, grandmother, nurturing caregiver. Although this trend has changed significantly, our thinking and practice lag far behind. The obvious implication is that as long as marriage and the nuclear family are touted as the only route for women, those who do not choose such a path will continue to be invisible or to be seen as deviant. Lesbians know the latter all too well as evidenced by one dinner participant who remarked: "We have existed in invisibility. I like the idea of being visible but I also think if there's a backlash against plain old feminism, what will the backlash be against lesbianism?" Another woman related this comment to her anticipatory fears about old age: "Sometimes I don't feel very optimistic that I'm going to be doing anything different when I'm 80, than being out when it's safe and not out when it's not safe."

Women's lives are not socially or culturally constructed to be fulfilling without men and/or children. The apparatus of the state, hand-in-hand with the family ethic depends on our partnership in marriage, on our mating with the opposite sex, of our reproducing the next generation. It is still assumed, for example, that when women reach midlife the major events are that our children may be ready to leave home, we may be entering the workforce, coping with menopause, or going back to school. Obscured are those who have always had waged work; who do not have children, who are not heterosexual. Yet, we are also women coping with menopause, we are also women from the early "boomer" years being admitted to universities and programs which were not accessible to us in our youth, and also perhaps among those watching our children leave home. Many of the midlife transitions lesbians face parallel those of married, divorced or widowed women–possible career change, health concerns, caretaking aging parents and/or other family members, the deaths of lovers, family and friends, and so on.

For decades feminist voices have been raised in support of alternatives for women. By merely being single, women challenge institutions that have set aside particular roles for them. Lesbians take that challenge even further by relating and choosing women as primary partners, friends, and lovers. Modleski (1991) argues that

> feminism has emphasized from the beginning the oppressiveness of the ideology of compulsory heterosexuality and the institution it supports–that of the nuclear family. The family is the structural unit keeping women economically and physically dependent on men; separating women from other women; and, in extreme (but by no means uncommon) cases, providing space in which men may abuse women with impunity. The special difficulties faced by lesbians under such a system are analogous to those of a prisoner who has escaped incarceration and, being 'at large,' faces more extreme punitive measures than many of the more docile inmates. The hazards faced by lesbians cannot be overestimated. (p. 13)

The much-quoted statistic informs us that between ten and twelve percent of the population is gay or lesbian. If this is the case, then the number of lesbians "at large" among the elderly population in Canada is considerable, and it will be necessary to break through fears and stereotypes that attach to women who remain outside the dominant vision. In order to increase our understanding of the experience of lesbian passages, it would be helpful to begin to re/image our situations since as Nicole Brossard (1988) has said of lesbians, we make ourselves up as we go along.

If we are seen or imagined, however, our image is read as deviant or inverted. Warland (1991) asks lesbians, "Why reclaim the word invert?" She responds that she is "attracted to the way the very word itself indicates a radically different position from which we see, experience and speak life–that it's not simply a matter of 'sexual preference'. . . . *Invert. To Turn.*

bend. Shape changers . . . " (p. xi). Renaming or reclaiming words about our lives, and inverting the way we image the world through *our* eyes, enables us to begin to imagine ourselves. We image ourselves in the public spaces of the world, and it is dangerous. Warland, a lesbian poet whose work plays with and inverts the dominant-tongue suggests:

> As a queer culture, we are not rooted in a particular geographical location; as lesbians we have not been able to preserve much of our history and art; and as dykes we are part of other cultures and races with profound differences among them. (p. xi)

Mainstream culture has difficulty exchanging its image of woman–it seems to have one image of her. She is a white fantasy woman. An imaged woman constructed over time from fragments of myth, film, television, from music videos, fashion magazines, children's toys, fairy tales. Certainly her image is not lesbian. Lesbian is invisible, or she is fractured–her image constructed from other deviant cultural and religious fragments that tend, or intend, to silence her naming of her life. The image, of course, is never an old woman. When many images of old women continue to parody and portray non-sexual "little old ladies," what becomes of women who have been primarily defined by their "deviant" sexuality, and who have been ascribed the frightening and tainted image of "lesbian"? Apprehension and fears of invisibility, current and future health and financial problems, and grappling with notions of community, are pivotal. One participant in our group commented that,

> If you're a lesbian and go into old age alone, you have to pretend you're a straight person, or as someone asexual. There's an assumption that you're heterosexual. It's a concern of mine that in my old age I'm going to be thrown into these institutions that serve straightness.

Lesbians warrant little, if any, attention in mainstream culture. Rather than portraying often self-sufficient women with "regular" lives–jobs or careers, possibly an intimate long-term relationship, social networks of friends and perhaps family and pets, the very word represents women to be feared/loathed because of their non-attachment to men. Why don't studies/practices take us into account? Cruickshank (1991) argues that, "In addition to the fact that the elderly population includes gay people, most mainstream gerontologists seem unaware of the small body of work produced by gay gerontologists . . . " (p. 77). It wasn't until 1979, for example, that the first major study of older American lesbians was undertaken. It is important to note that there may be unique ascriptions to aging lesbians. As Cruickshank suggests:

> Probably most middle-aged and old lesbians and gay men were told at some point in their lives that being gay was disastrous because they were certain to be lonely and pitiable in their old age. This message was a powerful social control that coerced many into marriage. Its persuasiveness came partly from ageism. Now that more positive images are beginning to appear, gay people can develop more realistic expectations of what the future holds, and gerontologists both mainstream and gay, can better understand the population they serve. (p. 86)

In the face of this, it seems crucial to document the everyday work of being a lesbian; and, the relationship between our invisible "presence," and the construction of lesbianism by a society that refuses our existence. It is imperative to chronicle the effort which goes in to constructing and maintaining a life in the face of stigma–a life often outside normative constructions of family, religion, community. To do this we continue to talk informally with lesbians in their forties, fifties and older, not in order to garner further experiences about our passages through midlife, or to elicit comparisons with heterosexual women, but rather to mull over and examine our experiences within the political, social and cultural context in which we live our lives. The women we have been speaking with are well aware of the aging process in their own lives. Aging is considered a challenge and each woman's experience of herself has shifted during midlife. While aging is a significant experience, and is considered a major turning point, some say they find the world a more comfortable place. Most feel more accepting of themselves and more self-assured, while others have absorbed some of society's preoccupation about youth: "I don't worry so much about what I look like although it's shocking to me. When I look in the mirror I don't see what I expect to see and it always surprises me that I really look like that."

In attempting to reconcile one's invisibility as lesbian women growing older, it is evident in our discussions that some lesbians have connections in multiple communities–whether they be communities of class, race, spirituality, arts or profession. Most of the lesbians we talked with are political and part of a larger lesbian feminist community and culture, yet they express ambivalence about it being an isolated or self-sufficient community, since it provides access to only one part of their lives. On the other hand, there is pressure not to create community, to maintain ourselves in/visibly, to unwittingly support and construct institutions that keep us separate. One dinner participant noted:

> We buy into the way everybody else does things. Society really pushes us to be fragmented and we take that on. As much as we talk about community, everything in the world works against it. We think it's us. It's a bigger issue and we can't succeed until we name it.

The issue is a difficult one. Will women with health problems, for example, be cared for by their families of origin, or by the lesbian community? Many hospitals and facilities do not allow lesbian partners as family. How is it possible to form community or to care for one another when there is no recognition of relationship whatever its context, and simultaneously work against the forces that counteract development of our own communities? A theme throughout our conversations has also been the fact that as lesbians we are disempowered because we are not a community in the way many of us would like. We are beginning to address how society and its institutions "push us to be fragmented," and to remain isolated as we age, more so than when we were younger. While there is some agreement about the importance of the lesbian community, the difficulty becomes how to create community that will nurture and provide for us when we are unable to care for ourselves. We are not immune to the influences of mainstream society and its reverence for the nuclear family. As one 45 year old woman remarked: "Despite having a different consciousness we're still taking care of our *unit* whether it's one or two." However, another woman noted that many of us have difficulty seeing ourselves in committed relationship–an aspect which will affect our old age: "In effect it's like two single people living together–we're not coupled the way straight people are"; like the mainstream world imagines us, many of us cannot see ourselves as family.

As with many women, lesbians too are surprised to discover that we have internalized the myth that we would be taken care of. To reach one's forties or even fifties and realize that you are the one who will need to continue providing for yourself often comes as a surprise even when you have always supported yourself. Confronting this myth is a painful realization for women whose health is in jeopardy now. As one woman told us, "I never thought I'd be debilitated in my forties. I feel like I'm a failure. I feel separated from and alienated from life." When her friends suggested she get support through the cancer clinic, she responded, "it would be like going to Mars. Nobody there has a lifestyle like I had . . . or have." She recognizes that institutions have been constructed with particular ill people in mind; an aging lesbian with cancer would not fit.

Thus, a major contradiction for midlife and aging lesbians with health problems *is* the concept of community. To whom can we/they turn? Often experiences with the health care system are not hers alone. Similar to documented reactions of many health care workers to persons with AIDS (Herringer, in press), lesbians in need of care are scrutinized, found undeserving, and refused care in subtle or overt ways. In particular, older lesbians feel unsafe and believe that social service and health professionals can "make a lot of trouble for us." Those of us who have been hospitalized during our younger adulthood know all too well from personal experience that the "system" does not take kindly to difference and diversity. One woman said, "they withheld my pain medication once they realized that she was my partner," while another woman noted that: "we told them we were sisters, and they thought it was so nice that we were such a close family." Our participants expressed considerable fear about the vulnerabilities of old age considered in light of these experiences.

As we grow older, the fear of poverty through illness or loss of employment is a vivid possibility regardless of whether or not we are in relationships. None of us wants to depend on family or be forced to rely on institutions where our safety is in jeopardy because we are lesbians. None of us wants to be invisible. Nonetheless, we exist in the underground, not the foreground. In the aging process we are only now making tentative attempts to name our strengths and limitations, to articulate our desires and fears to ourselves, to challenge the dominant image or construction of women that exists inside, as well as outside, each of us. It is apparent that we are only beginning to define our experiences to ourselves, and that our invisibility to ourselves parallels our invisibility in the larger society.

Says one poet, "I had no place to go . . . to hear a lesbian voice. How have we ever found each other? For a long time we sought each other only through the wordless look: searching for the other woman who was also looking, *really looking at you,* and seeing you, the woman who was the only lesbian. For a long time there were no public words for us" (Pratt, 1991, p. 30). Pratt's words highlight the need to make visible what happens when a woman makes herself the subject of her own gaze, or when she turns her gaze toward another woman. We must define ourselves. We must re/present ourselves. If we don't, we can be "made up," constructed by others, made to be object. When we begin to peel back layers of what it means to be a lesbian, to call ourselves lesbians, what holds the most meaning is what the image represents in the eyes of society. It does not matter what we have done in the past, suddenly we are seen only as our sexual practices. We are dismissed because of our bodies; and that is a measure of the threat we face. We are with and for women; consequently, as younger lesbians we lose our children, at any age we may lose our jobs, our housing and sometimes our lives. It becomes difficult or impossible to participate in communal ritual or religion. We are banished from convents, and, along with gay men, cannot minister in most churches.

When lesbians speak of our lives others often recoil or grow angry. Why do you have to name yourself a lesbian? Why do you have to call yourself anything? In that naming or making visible there are risks and many stay hidden. Some hide by themselves or with a lover; some pass, and wouldn't be recognized. Lesbians growing older, like their younger counterparts, like their heterosexual counterparts, are not the same. We share one commonality, however–the oppressive power of institutions that occasionally speak of differences but cannot welcome or even tolerate diversity. It would seem that any lesbian speaking out and placing her foot firmly on the earth is reworking her own image for herself and her communities. As Nicole Brossard (1988) argues, "a lesbian who does not reinvent the world is a lesbian in the process of disappearing."

REFERENCES

Auger, J. (1990). Lesbians and aging: Triple trouble or tremendous thrill. In S.D. Stone (Ed.). *Lesbians in Canada*. Toronto: Between the Lines.

Bishop, A. (1994). *Becoming an ally: Breaking the cycle of oppression*. Halifax: Fernwood Press.

Brossard, N. (1988). *The aerial letter*. Translated by M. Wildeman. Toronto: Women's Press.

Cruickshank, M. (1991). Lavender and gray: A brief survey of lesbian and gay aging studies. In J.A. Lee (Ed.). *Gay midlife and maturity*. Binghamton: Harrington Park Press.

Gallagher, K.A. (1996). Centering the margins: What can be learned from listening to the voices of lesbians over 55? Unpublished Master of Social Work Thesis: University of British Columbia.

Gee, E. M., & Kimball, M. M. (1987). *Women and aging*. Toronto: Butterworths.

Giele, J.Z. (Ed.). (1982). *Women in the middle years*. New York: John Wiley and Sons.

Herringer, B. (1991). Out of the Mainstream: Contemporary Canadian spinsters speak out. Paper presented at the Canadian Association on Gerontology Conference. Toronto.

Herringer, B. (1996). A clash of knowledge(s): Toward an analysis of the social organization of AIDS 'suicide'. *Canadian Social Work Review. 13* (1), 39-52.

Hufton, O. (1984). Women without men: Widows and spinsters in Britain and France in the eighteenth century. *Journal of Family History. 9*(4), 355-376.

Isaac, B., & Herringer, B. (1996). Pinking the Ivories: Academic outings in social work. *Canadian Woman Studies. 16* (2), 73-76.

Jeffreys, S. (1985). *The spinster and her enemies: Feminism and sexuality 1880-1930*. London: Pandora Press.

McCannell, K. & Herringer, B. (1990). Changing terms of endearment: Women and families. In J. Turner (Ed.). *Living the changes*. Winnipeg: University of Manitoba Press.

McCannell, K., McCarthy, C. & Herringer, B. (1992). Images of women in Canadian social policy: Em-bodying patriarchy. In D. Currie, and V. Raoul (Eds.). *Anatomy of gender: Women's struggle for the body*. Ottawa: Carleton University Press.

Modleski, T. (1991). *Feminism without women: Culture and criticism in "post-feminist" age*. London: Routledge.

Mullaly, R. (1993). *Structural social work: Ideology, theory and practice*. Toronto: McClelland & Stewart.

Neugarten, B. (1982). Middle age and aging. In B. Hess (Ed.). *Growing old in America* (2nd Ed.) New Brunswick, NJ: Transaction Books.

Pratt, M. B. (1991). When the words open into some not yet open space. In B. Warland (Ed). *Inversions: Writings by dykes, queers & lesbians*. Vancouver: Press Gang Publishers.

Simon, B. (1987). *Never married women*. Philadelphia: Temple University Press.

Vicinus, M. (1985). *Independent women*: *Work and community for single women 1850-1920*. Chicago: The University of Chicago Press.

Warland, B. (Ed.). (1991). *Inversions: Writings by dykes, queers & lesbians*. Vancouver: Press Gang Publishers.

Zone, J. S., Estes, C. L., & Binney, E. A. (1987). Gender, public policy and the oldest old. *Ageing and Society, 7*, 275-302.

Rural Lesbians' Strategies for Coming Out to Health Care Professionals

Kathleen A. Tiemann
Sally A. Kennedy
Myrna P. Haga

SUMMARY. The authors conducted in-depth interviews with lesbians from rural communities in the midwest about their interactions with health care professionals and how they decided whether to dis-

Kathleen A. Tiemann, PhD, is Associate Professor of Sociology at the University of North Dakota where she teaches classes on gender, research methods, introduction to sociology and women studies. Her research interests include lesbian studies, the mobility of departmental chairpersons in graduate departments of sociology and teaching sociology. Sally A. Kennedy, PhD, is a licensed psychologist, Adjunct Professor of Counseling Psychology and Staff Psychologist at the University of North Dakota Counseling Center. Her research interests include lesbian identity development and the impact of values on attitudes toward gays and lesbians. Myrna P. Haga, PhD, BCD, is Associate Professor of Social Work at the University of North Dakota. Her research interests include the experiences of lesbians who live in rural environments, clinical decision making and dual relationships in social work practice.

Address correspondence to: Kathleen A. Tiemann, Sociology Department, P.O. Box 7136, University of North Dakota, Grand Forks, ND 58202-7136 (Internet: tiemann@badlands.nodak.edu).

The authors wish to thank the women who told their stories so that they could help other lesbians. Thanks also to Clifford Staples, Morten Ender, and the reviewers for their comments.

[Haworth co-indexing entry note]: "Rural Lesbians' Strategies for Coming Out to Health Care Professionals." Tiemann, Kathleen A., Sally A. Kennedy, and Myrna P. Haga. Co-published simultaneously in *Journal of Lesbian Studies* (The Haworth Press, Inc.) Vol. 2, No. 1, 1998, pp. 61-75; and: *Gateways to Improving Lesbian Health and Health Care: Opening Doors* (ed: Christy M. Ponticelli) The Haworth Press, Inc., 1998, pp. 61-75; and: *Gateways to Improving Lesbian Health and Health Care: Opening Doors* (ed: Christy M. Ponticelli) Harrington Park Press, an imprint of The Haworth Press, Inc., 1998, pp. 61-75. Single or multiple copies of this article are available for a fee from The Haworth Document Delivery Service [1-800-342-9678, 9:00 a.m. - 5:00 p.m. (EST). E-mail address: getinfo@ haworth.com].

close their sexual orientation to them. They described the protective strategies they used when seeking health care and the responses they received to the disclosure of their sexual orientation. The four primary protective strategies included screening, planned disclosure, unplanned disclosure and non-disclosure. Participants voiced concerns over rejection or retaliation by health care professionals and by other community residents if their sexual orientation became known, and that they would be unable to obtain safe, appropriate care given the limited availability of health care service providers in their region. *[Article copies available for a fee from The Haworth Document Delivery Service: 1-800-342-9678. E-mail address: getinfo@haworth.com]*

If lesbians are often difficult to see (Eliason & Randall, 1991; Eliason, Donelan & Randall, 1992; Hitchcock & Wilson, 1992; Robertson, 1992), then rural lesbians are even more "invisible." Because of this invisibility, rural health care practitioners may not realize that they have lesbian patients and, as a result, they may be unprepared to meet lesbians' health care concerns. Moreover, because doctors, nurses and other helping professionals often accept the same stereotypes about lesbians that are held by the general public (Stevens, 1992), they may unwittingly create a situation in which lesbians are unable or unwilling to speak about themselves and their health care needs (Falco, 1991; Harris, 1996; Noble, 1996; Potter, 1985; Raboy, 1996; Rankow, 1996; Tiemann, Kennedy & Haga, 1997; Waitkevicz, 1996). In this article, we provide lesbians from rural areas with the opportunity to describe their experiences with members of the health care community and the protective strategies they used during these interactions.

PARTICIPANTS AND METHOD

A nonrandom sample of 8 rural lesbians was recruited by the investigators and by a student who knew lesbians who might be interested in participating in this research project. Five of the women lived in communities of fewer than 8,000 residents. However, these towns were within 80 miles of a "large" city of 50,000 people where the other three women lived. All had sought, and reported on, health care services they had received from providers who practiced in this city of 50,000 people.

It is important to recognize that the term "rural" does not simply refer to areas that are sparsely populated; there is a *gemeinschaft* that is shared by rural residents. To live in a rural community means that people believe that their neighbors share their values and way of life. Moreover, because their social spheres overlap, rural residents know who their neighbors are and much of what they do. This creates a paradox. On the one hand, because rural residents take for granted that their neighbors are just like them, differences often go unrecognized because they are not expected. On the other hand, when differences are intentionally or unintentionally revealed, it is a serious matter.

Those who do not conform to the norms of the rural community, like lesbians, face predictable sanctions. They are gossiped about, shunned, ostracized, encouraged to leave, and they may face acts of violence. Thus, to protect themselves and to keep their sexual orientation from becoming their master status, lesbians may try to remain closeted and, therefore, "invisible." All of the lesbians in our study were well aware of this rural *gemeinschaft* and had felt its effects on their lives.

Interviews were scheduled by phone for times and locations that suited the participants. All interviews were audiotaped and lasted between two and one-half to four hours. Participants provided detailed information about coming out, identity development, family interactions, health care experiences, and other issues. Here we focus exclusively on their interactions with physicians, therapists, counselors and psychiatrists.

Each interview was transcribed and health care stories were highlighted in the transcripts. After all of the health care stories were highlighted, the content and context of the stories were analyzed so that similarities and differences in reported experiences could be discerned. It was from this process that the four strategies of coming out to health care providers emerged.

At the time the interviews were conducted, the participants ranged in age from their early 20's through their mid-40's. Five women were in committed lesbian relationships of 8 to 18 years, two were partnered with women for 1 to 7 years, and one woman was single but dating. Two respondents had children. One woman and her lesbian partner chose to have a child together while the other woman had a child during her heterosexual marriage. These women were well educated: four had bachelors degrees, three had masters degrees or its equivalent, and one respondent was a full-time college student. The student held a part-time job and the other participants were employed full-time in professional and managerial occupations appropriate to their level of education. Despite their occupational levels, the median yearly income was $24,000 with a range from $10,000 to $50,000.

COMING OUT TO HEALTH CARE PROFESSIONALS

Lesbians, like their heterosexual sisters, need preventive and curative health care. However, they may have unique health care concerns and needs which are not met in a health care system that assumes all patients are heterosexual (Harris, 1996; Lucas, 1992; Noble, 1996; Raboy, 1996; E.J. Rankow, 1995; L. Rankow, 1996; Stevens, 1995; Tiemann et al., 1997; Trippet & Bain, 1992; Waitkevicz, 1996). Furthermore, they may deal with practitioners who are less knowledgeable than they are (Stevens, 1992; Stevens, 1995; Waitkevicz, 1996) or who pathologize their lesbianism and ignore the health care need that caused them to seek help (Hall, 1994; Stevens, 1992; Tiemann et al., 1997).

Some lesbians do not reveal information about their sexual orientation to health care professionals for fear of rejection, ridicule, disrespect and inappropriate treatment (Stevens, 1992; Stevens, 1994; Trippet & Bain, 1992). These are not idle fears. Stevens (1994) reported that the health care interaction stories told by lesbians from San Francisco were overwhelmingly negative. They felt unsafe, fearful and vulnerable in health care facilities and were sometimes treated disrespectfully. If it was difficult and dangerous for lesbians to disclose their sexual orientation to health care professionals given the relative anonymity provided in urban areas, how difficult must it be to make this disclosure for rural lesbians?

Health care professionals should assume that they will come into contact with sexual minority clients during their careers (Falco, 1991; Trippet & Bain, 1992) and that clients will be at different stages of self-acceptance as lesbian, gay, bisexual or transgendered people (Coleman, 1982; Falco, 1991; Hammersmith & Weinberg, 1973). Urban lesbians who came out to health care practitioners in one study were reportedly more comfortable with their sexual identity than those who did not come out. However, once they revealed their sexual orientations, they had "feelings of being 'exposed,' 'embarrassed,' and 'less anonymous' and of a 'void' in the relationship" (Robertson, 1992 p. 160). It is vital for health care professionals to provide a positive response when a client discloses her sexual orientation. Doing so not only helps a patient accept herself and her sexual orientation (Falco, 1991; Fassinger, 1991; Gentry, 1992; E.J. Rankow, 1995), but it may help create an environment in which she is more likely to seek routine health care in the future (Gentry, 1992; Stevens, 1992; Stevens & Hall, 1990).

PROTECTIVE STRATEGIES

The ways the rural lesbians in our study disclosed their sexual orientation to health care professionals varied, although there were four main protective strategies. The four strategies that emerged through content analysis of transcribed interviews were "screening," "unplanned disclosure," "planned disclosure," and "non-disclosure." These protective strategies are similar to those reported by Stevens (1994) and by Hitchcock and Wilson (1992) in their studies of multiethnic and socio-economically diverse lesbians in San Francisco. However, the lesbians we interviewed perceived higher risks and costs associated with the use of particular protective strategies. Because negative attitudes about lesbians and gays are normative in rural locales (Herek, 1991), being a known lesbian is potentially hazardous to one's health.

Screening

The first strategy used by our participants is "screening." The goal in screening is to locate a health care practitioner who is sensitive to lesbians and knowledgeable about their health care needs in the event that they intentionally or accidentally disclose their sexual orientation. This technique is most effective when seeking routine health care as there is time to do adequate research (Stevens, 1994).

Women who screen use two main techniques. One is to gather information about other lesbians' experiences with a particular health care worker before making an appointment. This, of course, is chancy as it means coming out and seeking contact with the lesbian community. For example, "Jody" said, "I've always scoped them out . . . so I really haven't ever had bad experiences with mental health professionals." "Tina" was more specific when she said that she and her lesbian friends talk to each other about which practitioners are "safe" to see and which ones are not.

A second means to locate a safe health care professional is to ask for a referral from a health care provider who is lesbian-friendly. For example, when "Mary" needed a new physician, she asked her psychiatrist for a referral. "Marsha," a helping professional herself, not only emphasized the importance of checking out health care providers to ensure safe and appropriate care, but had some advice for health care practitioners who believe that they do not have any gay or lesbian clients. She said,

> It must be because . . . people perceive you as not being sensitive . . . It might be to your advantage to get some counseling . . . or to educate yourself . . . [on] diversity issues . . . We won't share with you unless we feel safe . . . It's . . . your professional responsibility to do so.

"Laura" has had negative interactions with many health care professionals, but particularly with mental health professionals. She now carefully screens all of her health care providers and advocates an aggressive approach toward mental health practitioners who are unqualified to work with lesbian clients because of their hostility and lack of knowledge about lesbians and their lives. As she put it,

> The bad therapist should be outed . . . The problem is that you have to be in a community . . . to hear that information . . . I wish the APA would get really tough on regulating some of these assholes out of it.

As Laura noted, lesbians in rural areas, like their heterosexual counterparts, might be unaware of the lesbian community around them and the support and assistance it might provide. The "invisibility" of the lesbian community is enhanced by the fact that lesbians are not distinguishable from other women unless they choose to reveal their sexual orientation (Eliason et al., 1992; Eliason & Randall, 1991; Hitchcock & Wilson, 1992; Robertson, 1992). Marsha elaborated on that point when she said,

> There's a whole culture out there that I wasn't aware of . . . In a rural setting you don't know where it is. It's not plastered out there for the world to see.

Participants commented on the isolation they face in rural communities and how locating or establishing a lesbian community in these areas was risky. According to Laura,

> We don't have the community support [because] it's not as large a group of gay or lesbian people . . . You can't very well have much [of] a support group or anything else going on when there's like two of ya for how many miles . . . Everybody is so closeted anyway because they're so scared of getting beat up that they don't want to talk about it. So then you're even closeted to people of your own kind.

Therefore, even if a lesbian locates the lesbian community, she may be unsure of how to join it or she may fear reprisals for doing so. The limited visibility of and access to the lesbian community in rural areas cuts some lesbians off from important information about health care practitioners and from a social support system that could help them cope with health care concerns and with other problems of living.

A problem that all rural residents share is limited access to appropriate health care professionals in their region. Jody illustrated this problem when she noted that there were only three psychiatrists from which she could choose. This difficulty is compounded for a lesbian as she may have to make difficult choices about her health care needs. She may ignore a health care concern (Potter, 1985); if she can afford it, she may drive long distances for treatment from a sympathetic and knowledgeable practitioner, go to a health care provider who is uninformed about lesbian health issues or who treats her disrespectfully (Potter, 1985; Stevens, 1992; Stevens, 1994), rely on informal help from family or friends (D'Augelli, 1989; D'Augelli & Hart, 1987); or she may pursue health care locally but hide her sexual orientation as she does so (Hitchcock & Wilson, 1992; Potter, 1985; Stevens, 1994).

While they are not without risk, the screening strategies described by our participants increase the probability that a lesbian will receive a positive response if she comes out to a health care professional because practitioners who are known to be unsupportive, hostile or unqualified to treat lesbians are avoided whenever possible. Screening, in one of its forms, was used by everyone we interviewed even if they did not intend to disclose their sexual orientation. The heavy reliance on screening may be a result of the high level of education attained by our subjects. Those with less formal education may feel unable to successfully use this strategy. Nonetheless, screening is a protective strategy that helped lesbians feel safer when dealing with an often unfriendly health care community.

Unplanned Disclosure

Unplanned disclosure, the second strategy used by the lesbians in this study, was rather risky. Patients did not intend to reveal their lesbianism to their health care provider; their disclosure was prompted by a triggering event during their visit. Women who made unplanned disclosures reported a range of responses from health care practitioners. However, even the most favorable responses were inadequate. Marsha's story illustrates a common type of inappropriate response that some lesbians face when they make an unplanned disclosure of their lesbianism to a health care professional. Marsha made an appointment with a neurologist because she had severe headaches, memory losses, and lost track of time for 10 or 15 seconds. While taking her medical history, the neurologist asked Marsha why she did not use birth control:

> I thought, "Well, hell. I'll give this a try and see what happens." I said, "I'm a lesbian." From that point on his treatment of me was completely different. And he immediately decided that I should take the MMPI . . . [and that] a clinical psychologist should see me . . . His physical exam of me was so sloppy! . . . The minute I mentioned I was a lesbian then it was all over with. He did not entertain my

> symptoms as being valid at all. Everything that was wrong with me was because I was a lesbian. And I got up and I said, "I'm sorry. I don't need to be treated this way" and I walked right out.

Marsha took a calculated risk with her disclosure especially since this doctor was one of only two neurologists in the area. To Marsha's dismay, the result of her honesty was an inappropriate response from the doctor. Marsha responded as she did because she is a well-educated woman and a health care professional. A less informed patient may not have responded so assertively in these circumstances. As Marsha discovered after seeking assistance elsewhere, her symptoms were caused by a classic case of spinal compression; they were not due to her lesbian identity nor did she need mental health care.

Like Marsha, Jody made an unplanned disclosure of her sexual orientation. She described an "incredibly funny" incident with her allergist which further portrays the heterosexism and the stereotypes about lesbians that seem to flourish among some members of the medical community.

> He was going on and on about yeast infections . . . and I finally just said, "Dr.–, I'm a lesbian." And he said, "Oh, my dear. You know you are really a very good looking woman." . . . And he was going to give me a shot for it! He figured it [lesbianism] was part of a yeast allergy. And he thought it would "take care of my social problem as well," is the way he put it. I said, "You know, I really don't regard it as a problem." "Oh!" he said . . . I kinda knew he was like that . . . A few years prior . . . I wouldn't have told him.

Jody saw a practitioner that she knew had unconventional ideas before making an appointment because she knew what kind of health care she needed. Despite his "understanding" of the etiology of lesbianism, his belief in the stereotype that lesbians are unattractive, and his opinion that a lesbian sexual orientation can be converted into a heterosexual one through injections (and that alcoholics can be "cured" in a similar way), he is considered eccentric, but competent. Jody's experience may be unusual, but the lack of information among health care providers about lesbians and how their sexual orientation may affect their reason for seeking treatment is not (D'Augelli, 1989; D'Augelli & Hart, 1987; Falco, 1991; Stevens, 1992; Trippet & Bain, 1993).

Not all of our respondents reported unfavorable responses from physicians when they disclosed their sexual orientation. Mary's spontaneous disclosure of her sexual orientation to her female physician was one of the more positive ones reported by our subjects. Mary said,

> She's asking about all the risk factors for cervical cancer . . . and instead of trying to lie, I said, "I'm a lesbian." [She said,] "That's neat. Are you in a relationship?" She seems to have some information about lesbians . . . It's like some people don't . . . have to . . . think about how they're going to respond so that they can seem like they're okay with who you are.

While "that's neat" is a more positive response than those reported by Marsha, Jody or other participants, it still leaves much to be desired. Why is Mary's lesbian identity neat? Is it because Mary trusted her physician enough to disclose this information? Is it because the doctor expected to be educated about lesbianism by Mary, or is it neat for some other reason? While this response is more affirming than those that many lesbians receive from health care practitioners, it is still inadequate and troubling.

All of the women in our study who made unplanned disclosures of their sexual orientation to female physicians received positive reactions. However, the responses from male physicians were uniformly negative. The correlation between the sex of the health care provider and the type of response they gave to patients who disclosed their sexual orientation is consistent with reports offered by more diverse samples of urban lesbians (Hitchcock & Wilson, 1992; Stevens, 1994; Trippet & Bain, 1993). However, unlike their urban counterparts, rural lesbians have fewer health care professionals from which to choose if they encounter one who responds negatively to disclosure of their sexual orientation. The negative responses of male physicians reported here and elsewhere shed light on women's preferences for knowledgeable female health care providers over male health care professionals regardless of their sexual orientation (Stevens, 1992; Trippet & Bain, 1990; Trippet & Bain, 1993).

Planned Disclosure

The third strategy, planned disclosure, was used by women who felt that it was either necessary or desirable to reveal their sexual orientation to a health care practitioner. Like those who relied on screening, women who planned to disclose their sexual orientation gathered information about the health care professional so that they could determine how she or he might respond when they disclosed their sexual orientation. Some screening activities were completed before they made an appointment. Indeed, making an appointment was often dependent upon the results of what they learned. Other information could only be gathered while in the waiting room and during the woman's interaction with the health care provider.

The physical environment of an office or clinic can make clients feel at ease. Many of our participants mentioned how difficult it was for them to feel safe or accepted when office decorations and informational pamphlets were restricted to depictions of intact, heterosexual, European-American families (E.J. Rankow, 1995; Stevens, 1995). They defined this as disrespectful of any client who did not fit this narrow categorization. Moreover, the phrasing of questions and the available response categories on intake forms were described as biased and inappropriate to describe these women's lives. There was no way, for example, to indicate that they had a same-sex partner and that they had some concerns that were not shared by heterosexual women.

The behavior of the staff when clients are present also affects clients' perceptions of safety. Laura reported how she heard staff members at one human service agency tell gay jokes to their colleagues. They were seemingly unconcerned about being overheard by clients who were in the waiting room. This incident created an unsafe environment for their clients in general, but was especially painful to Laura as a lesbian.

During the office visit, close regard was paid to what the health care professional did and to how she or he responded to the patient and to her questions. Attention to these details and her "gut feelings" during the interaction helped determine whether a client disclosed her sexual orientation. For example, Tina said that she sometimes began to tell a health care professional about her sexual orientation, but

> when I got the feeling . . . [that they didn't accept my sexual orientation] . . . I quit going to them. . . . I trust my gut and when my gut said this isn't right, I left.

Like Tina, Jody carefully studied her psychiatrist to determine how he would respond to the disclosure of her sexual orientation. She described how difficult it was for her when she came out to him even after seeing him twice a week for two years:

> I called him and said, "This is real important and I need to come in and talk to you." So he found a half hour slot for me . . . And so I sat down and . . . just blurted it out. I said, "I just didn't tell you . . . all this time." And he said, "Oh, Jody . . . You know we've wasted a lot of time." I said, "I guess so but I just really just couldn't tell you that." And he said, "Did you think that I would think differently about you?" And I said, "I guess not really, but that I would feel different, you know? I mean it was like I needed to get to a place myself where it was okay with me before I could tell you."

Jody's psychiatrist was supportive of her sexual orientation, but he also expressed disappointment that she took two years to disclose it to him. We cannot know if he reflected on whether his behavior kept Jody from disclosing her lesbianism earlier in their professional relationship. We also cannot know how keeping her sexual orientation secret affected the appropriateness of the care she received nor whether it has changed how Jody's psychiatrist interacts with his other clients. What is clear, however, is that her psychiatrist missed a crucial therapeutic issue at Jody's expense.

Women who embraced the protective strategy of planned disclosure proceeded with caution. Like their urban counterparts, they worried about how knowledge of their sexual orientation might affect their clinical treatment (Stevens, 1994). They were also concerned with how their lesbianism would be judged and how that judgment might affect future interactions with, and access to, this and other health care practitioners (Robertson, 1992), especially if this information was recorded in their files (Gentry, 1992; Lucas, 1992). These are significant concerns in rural communities where health care professionals know one another, the availability of practitioners is limited, and many people have access to clients' files.

Non-Disclosure

"Non-disclosure" comprised the fourth protective strategy used by the lesbians in our study. Some of the lesbians we interviewed took pains to hide their sexual orientation not only from their health care provider, but also from others with whom they regularly interacted. This decision is at least partly related to residing in a rural community. Six of the eight women specifically commented on the danger of being a known or suspected lesbian. According to "Carol," "When you're out in rural [state] you better not let everybody know you're a lesbian or you might get killed." Laura was so concerned about her safety that she did not have newsletters, magazines, books, or anything else that could be "incriminating" sent to her through the mail because:

> If somebody else reads it because they're nosy, and they will, you get 50 million questions . . . I've had violent crimes done to several friends of mine in [a larger town of 32,000]. They . . . [had] windows shot out of their cars, guys being beat up, things like this. That frightens me.

These safety concerns were generalized to the medical community by our subjects. Urban lesbians who participated in studies by Gentry (1992) and Lucas (1992) reported fear that their sexual orientation would be recorded in their medical files where anyone at the facility could read it. This concern takes on special significance in small towns where private matters may quickly become public knowledge. "Debra" commented on this.

> In an urban area you can kind of hide a little better . . . In a rural town, you can't really mind your own business because everyone knows everything you're doing.

"Cathy" also addressed this issue. She revealed how, as a college student who was struggling with her lesbian identity, she had to summon up her courage to call the local mental health center's hotline for information.

> All I was looking for was . . . a group or something like that. [The hotline staff] kept on trying to get me into help, and at that point it was even such a risk for me to make that phone call . . . Once you are out in a small rural area . . . word spreads and people think it's their right to let everybody know . . . [You may] literally be run out of the community.

When Mary temporarily lived in a town of a few hundred people, she put her safety concerns this way:

> If someone thought you were gay and you went to a bar, they'd shoot you . . . If you look at them wrong or if they thought you were coming on to their girlfriend, male or female, they'd pull their pistol out or they'd beat you. . . . You just need to be real low key.

These concerns for physical safety keep some lesbians from disclosing their sexual orientation and from seeking the support and information that is available through the lesbian community. Mary's many negative experiences with helping professionals and her fear of retaliation and mistreatment have made her leery of coming out to most health care providers. On the few occasions that she has disclosed her sexual orientation, it was preceded by extensive research. Even then she only disclosed her sexual orientation after many favorable interactions with a health care provider with whom she felt very safe.

In some cases, the health care provider facilitated the protective strategy of non-disclosure. Recall how Jody's psychiatrist ignored her sexual orientation until she brought it up two years after beginning work with him despite the fact that it affected the clinical treatment she received. Mary reported a similar situation. She saw a counselor at a college psychological services center when she was an undergraduate. While her counselor understood the importance of facilitating Mary's self-acceptance, she never addressed Mary's lesbianism.

> I was in my first [lesbian] relationship . . . I talked about . . . [it as] being special . . . but she never brought up . . . being lesbian . . . I'm sure she knew that I was lesbian long before I accepted it.

Like Jody, Mary saw no problem with her clinician's failure to address her sexual orientation. Indeed, she was appreciative that her counselor did not directly address her sexual orientation. Unfortunately, this therapeutic decision helped Mary deny both her social and her personal identity as a lesbian and its possible effects on her life, including her life-long problem with recurrent depression (Falco, 1991; Fassinger, 1991).

The protective strategy of non-disclosure had both costs and benefits for these women. While this strategy allowed some lesbians to seek the health care they needed without fear of reprisal, it also meant that they may not have received appropriate care. For example, when used with mental health professionals non-disclosure kept some lesbians from directly revealing their sexual orientation. As a result, their therapy may have been hindered. Non-disclosure required vigilance and extraordinary energy on their parts so that their actual sexual orientation was not inadvertently revealed to health care providers. Moreover, lesbians' fears of reprisal from other residents of the rural areas in which they lived, should their sexual orientation become known, kept them from seeking help from the lesbian community around them.

DISCUSSION

Coming out is not a single event; it is an ongoing process in the lives of lesbians. It is motivated by the need for self-validation, acceptance by others, to meet potential partners, by the need for medical intervention for health care concerns and for help with problems of living (Trippet & Bain, 1993; Potter, 1985). Disclosure of one's sexual orientation in a heterosexist medical system to homophobic health care professionals can have a detrimental effect on a woman's self-esteem, her future help-seeking behavior and on her physical safety (L. Rankow, 1996; Stevens, 1992; Stevens, 1995; Trippet & Bain, 1993). Similarly, not coming out and presenting an inaccurate self to others also has costs.

The rural lesbians we interviewed emphasized the importance of using protective strategies so that they could feel safe in their interactions with members of health care professions. They stressed that most helping professionals needed further education so that they could move beyond stereotypes about lesbians, provide appropriate responses to coming out, and so that they could adequately address lesbians' health care concerns. Participants also underscored the need for all health care professionals to reflect upon their feelings about lesbians, their ability to competently treat them in their practices, and their ability to effectively refer them to other practitioners.

The results of this study are not generalizable because of the methodological problems associated with sampling a population that is relatively "invisible." Additionally, our informants may be more homogeneous than those included in other studies on the basis of race and education. Indeed, their relatively high level of education may have enhanced their ability to effectively strategize about selecting health care practitioners and determining whether they could safely disclose their sexual orientation to them. These concerns notwithstanding, the stories these women told provide a glimpse into the health care concerns faced by lesbians who live in and seek medical care in rural communities.

REFERENCES

Coleman, E. (1982). Developmental stages of the coming out process. *Journal of Homosexuality, 7,* 31-43.

D'Augelli, A.R. (1989). Lesbian women in a rural helping network: Exploring informal helping resources. *Women and Therapy, 8,* 119-130.

D'Augelli, A.R., & Hart, M.M. (1987). Gay women, men, and families in rural settings: Toward the development of helping communities. *American Journal of Community Psychology, 15,* 79-93.

Eliason, M.J., & Randall, C.E. (1991). Lesbian phobia in nursing students. *Western Journal of Nursing, 13,* 363-374.

Eliason, M., Donelan, C. & Randall, C. (1992). Lesbian stereotypes. *Health Care for Women International, 13,* 131-144.

Falco, K.L. (1991). *Psychotherapy with lesbian clients: Theory into practice.* New York: Brunner/Mazel.

Fassinger, R.E. (1991). The hidden minority: Issues and challenges in working with lesbian women and gay men. *The Counseling Psychologist, 19,* 157-176.

Gentry, S.E. (1992). Caring for lesbians in a homophobic society. *Health Care for Women International 13,* 173-180.

Hall, J.M. (1994). Lesbians recovering from alcohol problems: An ethnographic study of health care experiences. *Nursing Research, 43,* 238-244.

Hammersmith, S.K., & Weinberg, M.S. (1973). Homosexual identity: Commitment, adjustment, and significant others. *Sociometry, 36,* 56-79.

Harris, A. (1996). The invisibility of lesbians with AIDS. In G. Vida (Ed.), *The new our right to love: A lesbian resource book* (pp. 108-111). New York: Touchstone.

Herek, G.M. (1991). Stigma, prejudice, and violence against lesbians and gay men. In J.C. Gonsiorek and J.D. Weinrich (Eds.), *Homosexuality: Research and implications for public policy.* Newbury Park, CA: Sage.

Hitchcock, J.M., & Wilson, H.S. (1992). Personal risking: Lesbian self-disclosure of sexual orientation to professional health care providers. *Nursing Research, 41,* 178-183.

Lucas, V.A. (1992). An investigation of the health care preferences of the lesbian population. *Health Care for Women International, 13,* 221-228.

Noble, R.E. (1996). Chemical dependency: The journey home. In G. Vida (Ed.), *The new our right to love: A lesbian resource book* (pp. 102-104). New York: Touchstone.

Potter, S. (1985). Social work, traditional health care systems and lesbian invisibility. *Feminist Perspectives on Social Work and Human Sexuality, 20,* 59-68.

Raboy, B. (1996). Getting pregnant through donor insemination. In G. Vida (Ed.), *The new our right to love: A lesbian resource book* (pp. 99-102). New York: Touchstone.

Rankow, E.J. (1995). Lesbian health issues for the primary care provider. *The Journal of Family Practice, 40,* 486-493.

Rankow, L. (1996). Breast and cervical cancer among lesbians. In G. Vida (Ed.), *The new our right to love: A lesbian resource book* (pp. 96-99). New York: Touchstone.

Robertson, M.M. (1992). Lesbians as an invisible minority in the health services arena. *Health Care for Women International, 13,* 155-163.

Stevens, P.E. (1992). Lesbian health care research: A review of the literature from 1970 to 1990. *Health Care for Women International, 13,* 91-120.

Stevens, P.E. (1994). Protective strategies of lesbian clients in health care environments. *Research in Nursing & Health, 17,* 217-229.

Stevens, P.E. (1995). Structural and interpersonal impact of heterosexual assumptions on lesbian health care clients. *Nursing Research, 44,* 25-30.

Stevens, P.E., & J.M. Hall. (1990). Abusive health care interactions experienced by lesbians: A case of institutional violence in the treatment of women. *Response: To the Victimization of Women and Children, 13,* 23-27.

Tiemann, K.A., Kennedy, S.A. & Haga, M.P. 1997. Lesbian's experiences with helping professionals. *Affilia, 12,* 84-95.

Trippet, S.E., & Bain, J. (1990). Preliminary study of lesbian health concerns. *Health Values, 14,* 30-36.

Trippet, S.E., & Bain, J. (1992). Reasons American lesbians fail to seek traditional health care. *Health Care for Women International, 13,* 145-153.

Trippet, S.E., & Bain, J. (1993). Physical health problems and concerns of lesbians. *Women & Health, 20,* 59-71.

Waitkevicz, H.J. (1996). Lesbian health issues. In G. Vida (Ed.), *The new our right to love: A lesbian resource book* (pp. 93-95). New York: Touchstone.

The Experiences of Lesbians of Color in Health Care Encounters: Narrative Insights for Improving Access and Quality

Patricia E. Stevens

Patricia E. Stevens, RN, PhD, is currently Associate Professor at University of Wisconsin-Milwaukee School of Nursing. In 1992, she received her PhD in nursing from the University of California, San Francisco. From 1992 to 1994, she was a Postdoctoral Fellow at University of California, San Francisco supported by a National Research Service Award Individual Postdoctoral Fellowship from the National Institutes of Health to conduct research about lesbians and HIV. Her continued research interests include lesbian health, primary and secondary prevention of HIV/AIDS in women, and narrative research with women who are living with HIV/AIDS. She has published widely about lesbian health, access to health care, women and HIV/AIDS, community-based HIV prevention, critical and feminist theories, and qualitative research methodology. She is a member of several editorial review boards of professional journals.

Address correspondence to: Patricia E. Stevens, University of Wisconsin-Milwaukee, School of Nursing, P. O. Box 413, Milwaukee, WI 53201.

This research was funded through a National Research Service Award Individual Predoctoral Fellowship from the National Institute of Nursing Research, National Institutes of Health #F31 NRO6323. The author gratefully acknowledges the women who so generously shared their health-care stories, the many community members who insured the successful completion of this project, her colleague, Joanne M. Hall, RN, PhD, for her steadfast scholarly insights, and Afaf Ibrahim Meleis, PhD, FAAN for her adept and challenging mentorship.

[Haworth co-indexing entry note]: "The Experiences of Lesbians of Color in Health Care Encounters: Narrative Insights for Improving Access and Quality." Stevens, Patricia E. Co-published simultaneously in *Journal of Lesbian Studies* (The Haworth Press, Inc.) Vol. 2, No. 1, 1998, pp. 77-94; and: *Gateways to Improving Lesbian Health and Health Care: Opening Doors* (ed: Christy M. Ponticelli) The Haworth Press, Inc., 1998, pp. 77-94; and: *Gateways to Improving Lesbian Health and Health Care: Opening Doors* (ed: Christy M. Ponticelli) Harrington Park Press, an imprint of The Haworth Press, Inc., 1998, pp. 77-94. Single or multiple copies of this article are available for a fee from The Haworth Document Delivery Service [1-800-342-9678, 9:00 a.m. - 5:00 p.m. (EST). E-mail address: getinfo@haworth.com].

SUMMARY. In this feminist narrative study, lesbians of color gave testimony to the effects of prejudice in face-to-face health care interactions. A major objective was to involve participants from a broad range of ethnic/racial backgrounds and socio-economic circumstances in open-ended interviews about their experiences receiving health care. Half of the 45 women in the sample were lesbians of color: 20% (9) African American, 18% (8) Latina, 11% (5) Asian/Pacific Islander, and 2% (1) Native American. Results suggest that if we wish to improve access to and quality of health services, those in the health care field must address race, class, gender, and sexual orientation prejudice in health care interactions, acknowledging the role discriminatory behavior plays in diminishing the availability of health care for lesbians of color. *[Article copies available for a fee from The Haworth Document Delivery Service: 1-800-342-9678. E-mail address: getinfo@haworth.com]*

How often have health care providers felt baffled by clients not seeking care in a timely fashion, resisting suggestions, and missing appointments? How troubled and perplexed might health care providers be to learn that they are not trusted by clients, that they are perceived to be part and parcel of an inhumane system? In health care encounters with members of marginalized populations, providers often feel frustrated, angry, and defensive about being viewed as "racist" or "classist" or "homophobic." Their standpoint on the situation may be that they are doing the best they can with all the structural impediments that intrude upon their interactions with clients. It is clients' experiences in these interactions, however, not providers' intentions or lack thereof, that influence whether clients even come back (Stevens, 1993).

The client-provider relationship is the core of the therapeutic alliance (Liaschenko, 1993), and determines to a large degree clients' access to health care (Stevens, 1994a). Yet little is known about how providers' behaviors influence clients' perceptions of safety and respect. It may be difficult for individuals who are socialized to be professionals to imagine the life circumstances of marginalized people in this society (Hall, Stevens, & Meleis, 1994). The day-to-day realities faced by women who are multiply stigmatized are often far from physicians' and other health care providers' mental grasp (hooks, 1984), especially in systems of care that demand a minimum of time spent with each client. The disparity in power and prerogative is likely little more than passing thought for busy clinicians, but can be acutely felt by clients (Stevens, 1996).

Although many providers may sincerely believe that they are open to clients' expressed needs and cultural diversity, the reality is that they often do not know how they are being perceived by marginalized clients, such as lesbians of color. Today's service delivery systems do not allow for clients to express their ideas and concerns freely, outside of preset, narrowly circumscribed diagnostic history-taking. With little access to clients' perspectives, providers are in a position of *not knowing what they do not know* about clients' experiences within the health care encounter. It is the existence of these blind spots that is particularly problematic. The smooth machinery of managed care is ill-fitted to externalizing clients' feelings and understandings. Clients' perceptions are either ignored or unwittingly passed over, until crises erupt, conflicts flare, or clients simply stop showing up. Clients may be traumatized by encounters with health care providers, and providers may learn nothing new from these situations, because communication wires are not intact.

Research like that reported here is essential for establishing some line of communication so that client experience can be known. The goal of this qualitative research, a feminist narrative study, was to document lesbians' experiences in health care from their perspective as clients. A major objective was to involve participants from a broad range of ethnic/racial backgrounds and socio-economic circumstances. The specific focus of this paper is to elaborate health care experiences described by lesbians of color. Half of the 45 women in the sample were lesbians of color. They related stories of their health care, positive and negative, providing a rich source of data about their perceptions of health care providers.

Narrative is a lens through which to study and convey women's experiences from a feminist perspective (Stevens, 1993). Significant life events are commonly communicated in story form, so narrative inquiry taps into people's everyday ways of expressing themselves (Riessman, 1993). Narratives incorporate the context and chronology of events while imparting the meanings they have for the storytellers. Stories, more than other forms of conversation, pull the listener into the teller's point of view. They draw the listener so deeply into the teller's experience that the listener can almost feel what it was like to be there.

METHOD

Sample

A total of 45 lesbians participated in this feminist narrative study in San Francisco; 32 were individually interviewed and 13 others were involved in 3 focus groups. Participants met the inclusion criteria: self-identified as lesbian, at least 21 years old, and conversant in English. Recruitment was accomplished through community-based purposive sampling (Biernacki & Waldorf, 1981). From the outset, a core of eight informants who were knowledgeable and influential members of African American, Latina, Asian/Pacific Islander, and Euro-American subgroups of the San Francisco lesbian community collaborated with me, a Euro-American lesbian researcher. They helped formulate research questions, devise sampling strategies, and validate findings. Their endorsement of the project, contacts with community members, and referral efforts were instrumental in recruiting a racially and economically diverse sample.

Half of the sample were women of color: 20% (9) African American, 18% (8) Latina, 11% (5) Asian/Pacific Islander, and 2% (1) Native American. The other 49% (22) were Euro-American. The mean age was 36, ranging from 21 to 56. The women were well educated: 69% (31) held college degrees. They worked in a variety of occupations, mostly in service sector categories (e.g., clerical work, unlicensed health work). The mean annual income was $26,000. Sixty-four percent (29) earned below the average annual pay in the San Francisco area (U.S. Department of Labor, 1991). Forty percent (18) reported chronic health conditions (e.g., hypertension, diabetes, immunocompetence disorders, cancer, orthopedic problems). Thirty-six percent (16) had no health insurance. All participants indicated that a circle of lesbian friends was primary to their social networks; only half named blood relatives as sources of support. Seventy-six percent (34) were in partnered relationships. Eighteen percent (8) had children. Eighty percent (36) were widely disclosed as lesbians.

Data Collection

I conducted the two-hour-long interviews most often in women's homes, sometimes in my home or at a lesbian community space such as a women's cafe. The focus groups, which were co-facilitated with an informant, occurred at the beginning, middle, and end of the data collection period, and were held at sites that housed lesbian community organizations. Each lasted about three hours. Upon meeting for interviews or focus groups, informed consent was obtained. All interviews and focus groups were audiotaped. I kept fieldnotes about the data collection, documenting environmental circumstances, participant characteristics, nonverbal behaviors, affect, communication processes, rapport, power dynamics, my impressions, and any problems (Briggs, 1986; Mishler, 1986). All procedures were approved by the Committee on Human Research at University of California, San Francisco.

I encouraged participants to tell stories, rather than answer standardized questions in a stimulus-response fashion. And I tried not to control the focus of conversation. I introduced broad topics and used reflexive, open-ended questions. I asked women: "What has it been like for you to get health care? I would like to hear about health care that has gone well for you and about health care that has not gone so well." This initial request was usually met with extensive storytelling. The lesbians in this study were eager to talk about what had happened to them in health care encounters. Sometimes an hour or more would pass before I inserted any follow-up questions because the women were so articulate in communicating the stories of their experiences in health care.

I did not interrupt women in the interviews. As Riessman (1987) suggests, women have multiple ways of narrating, and researchers need to respect their norms for telling stories. For instance, some women tell stories chronologically: this happened, then that happened. Others connect episodes by what they mean. They might tell what happened last month, then move to a story with a similar theme that occurred in their adolescence. If researchers keep interrupting women to get them to make their point or stay on the topic, stories cannot be told. By remaining silent at key points, I was able to actively listen as each participant paced the interview and developed its content. When necessary, I used probes and reflections to get more specific experiential detail, but I did so only after the initial telling of stories or when a participant indicated her desire for me to more directly structure the conversation.

At the end of interviews, I asked women for feedback about the research process. Generally, participants indicated that I conveyed genuine interest in their experiences and facilitated their comfort in disclosing by my lack of interruption, the open-ended nature of my questions, as well as the calm and expressiveness of my face, voice, and body language. I believe these interview tactics were successful in eliciting rich health care narratives because they: (1) did not disrupt participants' patterns of association regarding their experiences, (2) allowed participants to use their own words instead of dictating vocabulary, and (3) helped me, the researcher, to listen rather than give information. Regulating researcher domination in this way allowed participants the opportunity to talk about what was important to them, which increased the validity of the data.

Data Analysis

I transcribed verbatim the audiotapes of individual interviews, focus groups, and fieldnotes to create a textual database. Because of the storied nature of the data, I devised a multi-staged narrative analysis (Stevens, 1994a). The level of abstraction I sought did not forsake context. After listening to the tapes and reading through the transcriptions several times,

I was familiar enough to begin the formal analysis. The first stage was to demarcate boundaries of each story. Story was operationalized as the relating of a single interactional encounter in health care. Stories have recognizable beginnings, middles, and ends. They include the events that occurred and the interpretations placed on them by the teller. To designate text as story, specific structural elements were necessary: orientation, complication, evaluation, and resolution (Labov & Waletzky, 1967):

1. *Orientation:* a recognizable beginning made up of statements that have a referential function; telling person, place, time, or behavioral situation. Often these references precede story action; sometimes they are found throughout a story.
2. *Complication:* the main body of story action which is comprised of a series of events that are linked temporally or causally.
3. *Evaluation:* descriptions and elaborations that suspend the action and make meaning of the events. These statements establish the storyteller's point of view, indicate the relative importance of events, and show the storyteller's attitude toward what is happening, the persons involved, and the context of the story. Evaluative clauses constitute the "soul" of a story and are especially important because they convey the teller's understanding of what happened and why.
4. *Resolution:* a recognizable ending wherein results of the story are reported. The resolution may have a coda, which is a functional device for returning the verbal perspective back to the present moment (e.g., a story might end with a phrase like "And that was that.").

In this analytical process, 332 health care stories were demarcated and became the units of analysis. In other words, the 45 participants in the study related stories about 332 separate health care encounters. In stage two, each of the 332 stories was examined dialectically, that is, reported events as well as evaluations of those events were analyzed. I looked at the content of story events and what they meant to the storyteller. I constructed an adequate paraphrase (Polanyi, 1985) of each story to highlight the main plot and context of the action, persons involved, and participants' evaluations of story events. I paid attention in each case to the woman's pre-existing expectations and beliefs, environmental conditions of the health care encounter, unfolding events, and her interpretations and responses as the client.

The third stage involved looking at the positivity or negativity with which participants regarded each of their health care encounters. To adequately determine women's evaluations, both what they said and how they said it were examined. I consulted the transcripts for choice of vocabulary. I listened to the tapes for vocal intonation. And I referred to my fieldnotes for observations about body language. No story in this database was equivocally evaluated, in fact, there was a conspicuous certainty with which these women appraised the favorableness of their health care. There were only two types of evaluation. Either a health care encounter was positive or it was negative.

The fourth stage of analysis involved searching for story similarities and differences among individual participants and among ethnic/racial, socioeconomic, and health status subgroups in the sample. While distinguishing the diversity of health care circumstances and meanings across the differently situated individuals in the study, I also identified patterns of shared experiences (Richardson, 1988). Again a dialectic was set up whereby I explored the range and variability of individual experiences while also identifying collective realities.

Adherence to standards of rigor in feminist interpretive research, including dependability, reflexivity, credibility, coherence, consensus, and complexity (Hall & Stevens, 1991), substantiated the scientific adequacy of the project. As further demonstration of validity, I incorporate active voices of participants in this report to support analytic arguments. Pseudonyms are used.

RESULTS

Perceptions of Prejudice

The health care encounter stories of lesbians of color provide an insider's view of the health care landscape. As clients in health care interactions they were acutely aware of providers' behaviors and on many occasions interpreted what they saw and heard as signalling prejudicial assumptions on the part of health care providers. They were not talking about attitudes alone. Rather, they were saying that providers' assumptions are communicated in their behaviors. These behaviors may be overt; they may be subtle. Even when providers are not conspicuously discriminatory, their facial expressions, gestures, posture, words, and intonations can betray cautiousness, surprise, disapproval, and discomfort. As Opal, an African American lesbian mother, said:

- When doctors find out that I am lesbian, it throws them off pattern. They don't know how to adjust. They look startled or they gulp really hard or they start looking at the floor instead of at me. I guess it is so hard for them to lay aside their assumptions and look at me sitting there and realize that my life is a lot different from what they thought. They don't know what kinds of questions to ask or what subjects to talk about because they are so nervous. I think I lose a lot in the treatment, in the diagnosis, in the whole thing that I go in there for.

One woman used an analogy to describe her experience:

- Imagine you are in a women's restroom and a man walks in. What do the women in the restroom do? They look at the man like "What are you doing here?" There is a kind of a halt, like, "Whoa! What is going on here?" That is what it is like when a doctor or a nurse finds out that I am a lesbian.

I asked this participant what she might tell a room full of health professionals. She said she would pose this question:

- Have you ever felt uncomfortable around lesbians? If your answer is yes, do you think they didn't know that?

This statement is revealing in that the participant is aware that providers may not have considered the possibility that their discomfort around lesbians is perceptible. Yet providers' sudden "halt" in routine is very apparent to clients and is fitted within an experiential schema to reinforce a wariness lesbian clients tend to have, not only about the current provider, but probably about future ones as well.

Stories from participants of color in this study revealed that they perceived prejudice, not only about sexual orientation, but also about race, class, and gender, sometimes simultaneously. From her viewpoint, this is how Katherine, a 34 year old African American, saw it:

- White male doctors make it their job to see to it that Black women do not have any more babies. They lash out with a vengeance at every Black woman who comes to them, lecturing us about preventing pregnancy, giving us a real talking to. Whenever I went in, they would never let up when I said, no, I don't need birth control. So, sometimes I would come out as a lesbian, just to get them to move on to other things. The doctors would fumble around and say something like, "Oh . . . oh . . . I'm sorry." It was so awkward. . . . I always felt harassed because I am Black and because I am a lesbian.

In this case, a blind spot that many health care providers have, the assumption that all women are heterosexually active, was acted upon. As a result, Katherine felt forced into a disclosure of her lesbian identity and was discomforted by the response she got. But for this African American woman, the provider behaviors she described had an even deeper meaning. Her interpretations were tied to experiences of racism in which Black women's reproductive options are judged and monitored. She evidently faced this scenario time and time again, reinforcing her distrust of and anger with "white male doctors."

Exemplar story. To highlight the content of stories told by lesbians of color, I present an extended excerpt from Dinah's interview. Dinah was a 51 year old African American participant. The events she described stand out as paradigmatic in showing how women of color in the sample had to pay heed to a constellation of interactional dynamics in health care. Dinah's evaluations demonstrate that her identities as lesbian, woman, and African American were all salient in her understanding of what happened. This is the story she related in response to my opening question about what it had been like obtaining health care:

- I can tell you one experience that was really negative. It was what made me find the doctor I have now. It was 4 years ago. I had just been diagnosed with hypertension and then I had to change insurance policies because I got a new job. Well, I had this new HMO coverage and I knew I needed to get a complete physical exam. So I made an appointment. It was my first time going there. I saw this nurse practitioner. I liked her. I was really surprised by her response, her narrow-mindedness.

At this point, it is important to note that Dinah, the client, began with a positive impression of the provider, and was ready to invest her trust:

- She was doing a history on me and she was asking about pregnancies, so I thought it was a good time to tell her I was lesbian. When I said lesbian, it just took this nurse completely off guard. She started spelling it out loud as she wrote it in my chart, l-e-s-b-i-a-n. A nervous smile came over her face and she could not recompose herself. She left the room. I heard her talking to somebody in the hallway. And when she came back in, this other person was peering in at me from behind the door. I couldn't believe it was happening. There I was, half dressed. I was humiliated.

With this turn of events, Dinah's focus shifted from engaging in a dialogue with the nurse to an immediate sense of vulnerability. She was alarmed to realize that she had "undressed" emotionally and physically before someone who could not cope with her as who she was.

- At the end, the nurse told me to come back in a couple of weeks for a gynecological exam. She set me up to see what turned out to be this male doctor. His approach was so insensitive.

Dinah uses the words "set me up," perhaps because at this point in the interaction, she cannot trust the nurse. Evidently the nurse offered no explanation for her behavior or that of the person "peering" from behind the door. Given the totality of her experience, Dinah likely had little choice but to conclude that the nurse did not wish to see her again and with some level of intent "set her up" to see an "insensitive" male physician.

- As soon as I got in the room, a nurse's aide told me to get undressed and get up on the table. She left. Then he walked in. We had never met. He did not make any conversation with me. He was in the room one minute and he had that cold speculum in my vagina. I mean it happened just like that (snaps fingers). And I felt so intruded upon. I felt violated. Naturally I didn't say anything to him at that moment, laying there naked and everything.

Feeling even more vulnerable during this second encounter at the HMO, Dinah is quite aware that this time there is no conversation, no time to get to "like" the unfamiliar provider. The physician probably did not know about the difficulty the nurse's behavior posed for this client during her previous health care visit. He will also have a blind spot about how his speculum technique was perceived, because it so devastated Dinah that she was stunned and frightened, unable to speak.

- And what all came out was that, after I was dressed and I was out in the foyer, he gives me this slip of paper and says he wants me to go take another test. And I said, "What is this for?" And he said, "Syphilis." And I said, "Syphilis! Why are you testing me for syphilis? I don't have syphilis. I can't possibly have syphilis!'" He had taken one look at me and automatically ordered a syphilis test because I was a Black woman. Everything just went wild inside of me. There I was. I had just had an exam in which I felt violated as a woman. I already knew by what the nurse had done two weeks before, that being a lesbian was something they didn't like here either. Now to be treated like I was a reservoir for disease because I am Black. It was all wrong. I told myself, "I've got to get out of here."

This final interaction with the provider was not only insulting and annoying; it was *alarming*. As a whole, the series of events signalled *danger* from which she felt she had to escape.

- I could not go back there to that HMO. That is what made me know I had to get a new insurance plan and a new doctor.

Thus, Dinah brought the story full circle, completing the telling of the negative experience that made her find the doctor she sees now.

Effects of Prejudice: Fear and Foreclosed Options

Thematically, Dinah's story exemplifies many of those told by lesbians of color in the study. They described fears that prejudicial assumptions could affect the quality and safety of the health services they received. Helen, a 35 year old African American, talked about an incident in which all these fears came alive for her:

- I had to go to this specialist for a biopsy of my wrist. He was a straight, white male who was a stranger to me. He was exactly opposite of who I am and the first thing he said to me was, "I want you to trust me." That kind of opening made me feel fearful. History has taught me not to trust you. He started cutting and I saw blood running down my arm. I got scared and I said, "What's going on?" "Nothing," he said to me. I breathed my way through it. At one point I felt a twitching and I thought maybe he was cutting a nerve. Then my mind really started playing tricks. I began to have fantasies of the knife slipping and cutting off my left hand. I started thinking, What if some member of this guy's family was mugged by a Black person once? What if he had a fight with his wife this morning and he isn't feeling so kindly toward women today? Is he ethical enough to separate from all of that and not make it about me? Trust him, sure. We are asked all the time to trust that doctors are not carrying personal prejudices. Where is our guarantee of that?

The need to command the client to "trust" suggests that there is some reason why the client might not trust the provider. Furthermore, Helen had no information about what trust would mean in this situation: Don't move? This will hurt, but not much? You will see a lot of blood, but it is OK? I am white, but I will do the job correctly on a Black person? By the middle of the encounter, Helen was in great distress. Thoughts had intruded and she imagined that the actions of another member of her race may have angered the family of the provider at some point in the past, and now in retaliation, he might remove her limb. How ingrained and extensive must racism toward African Americans in the U.S. be to prompt this caliber of fear? Is it likely that the provider would suppose such thoughts were in the mind of this client during the biopsy he was performing? What changes in practice would be necessary to allay this level of fear?

Generally, women's fears came from concrete experiences as attested in their health care stories. Their narrations chronicled health care providers' slights as well as hostilities, their raised eyebrows as well as denigrations. Ella explained her perceptions in one encounter:

- The doctor had already made his mind up about what was wrong with me, a young Chicana woman. I tried to explain the pain I was having with what ended up being endometriosis. But he kept cutting me off with his questions about whether I had a job, what kinds of street drugs I used, where I lived. He had his own ideas about people like me and it didn't matter what I said.

Echoing Ella's experience, most of the women of color had stories to tell about health care incidents in which the most superficial cues about their appearance or language tapped into a well of assumptions about ethnicity/race:

- Doctors assume they know about me when they don't. They think I'm Jamaican because I have dreadlocks. They start talking to me about reggae music.
- When I ask an informed question, doctors get a startled look on their faces, like a Black woman isn't supposed to know enough to be able to ask that.
- My accent throws them off. Doctors and nurses assume I don't understand what they are saying. So they repeat over and over the simplest phrases and talk very loudly. It is very patronizing.

Irma, a 41 year old Puerto Rican, related this experience:

- At the HMO I used to go to they kept cancelling my appointments at the last minute without any regard for my work schedule. I asked around. I worked with seven other people who had that HMO and this never happened to any of them. When I finally got in, the doctor took one look at me and said, "Oh, I thought you were Hispanic." I wondered, Why are you making such a statement? Am I lighter skinned than other Latina women you have seen? Do I speak English more fluently? Does it seem odd to you that I am a professional? They see a name on the form and they expect a certain kind of person. And I inferred what he did not say, that because my surname is Hispanic, it is ok to cancel my appointments.

Racist and classist ideas seemed to reinforce each other to fuel health care providers' behaviors, as this participant narrates:

- My lover had surgery at the county hospital. She went in for the tests before the operation and a woman doctor she had never met before started talking about a hysterectomy. That was not what the surgery was supposed to be. And my lover got very upset. She tried to explain to the woman that she must be mistaken, that a hysterectomy was not what was supposed to be happening. And the doctor refused to believe her. She tried to turn it around, that my lover was the one who had misunderstood. The assumption was that my lover uses public services, she's poor, therefore, she is unintelligent. On top of that, she is African American, so that puts her in another category. She can't possibly be educated. Thank God, she made complaints and it got straightened out. And she received an apology. But what if she hadn't spoken up? Would she have gotten the wrong surgery?

In this case, a great deal of energy had to be expended to convince the provider that the client was correct, leaving the client and her lover doubting that low-income, African American lesbians can count on safe and competent care.

Shirley, a 36 year old African American lesbian mother without health insurance, related a similar experience with providers' disparaging presumptions about her intellectual capacities:

- There were some doctors who treated me and my kid who didn't talk to me, didn't explain what they were doing, didn't tell me what my kid had. They acted like I was dumb and they didn't want me to interfere. They talked down to me. I felt bad. I felt like they had put this box over me. Poor equals dumb. Poor equals uneducated. They were making all these assumptions about me. I felt forced to wear the box. I was too embarrassed to tell them I had a college degree and still had to use public services.

Shirley's comments indicate that to use the system to get the services that she and her child needed, she had to continually face providers' abrupt and silencing behaviors. She attributed these behaviors to prejudicial stereotyping of her race and low-income status. The fact that she worked a full-time job that provided little pay and no health benefits left her no choice but to use public services. Her resignation and shame made it difficult for her to protest "the box" she felt forced into.

These excerpts suggest that providers make oppressive associations among race, low income, and level of intelligence, resulting in women's alienation from and distress in health care contexts. A Euro-American participant's statements provide yet another example:

- Health care providers assume you are a minority if you are using the public system. Several times they have entered the room speaking Spanish to me. I am not Latina. It bothers me. Their assumptions are offensive because they are based on racism. I have had other providers over the years insist that I must be part Black. It mystifies me because I have very Anglo features. When you are poor they just automatically assume you must be a person of color.

Prejudicial assumptions had the potential to deprive clients of resources, adequate diagnoses, proper treatment, and personal dignity. Rosa, a 42 year old Puerto Rican woman with chronic asthma, told her story of trying to get SSI disability. The physician rejected her petition. He said, "If you weren't so lazy, you could get a job. This asthma of yours is psychological." Rosa was shocked and started to tell the doctor about her job history, that she had worked since she was 13 years old. He interrupted and said, "You people are all the same." Rosa was both humiliated and enraged by what she interpreted as a racist remark. She said, "They call me a lazy spic out on the streets, but why should I have to hear it in the doctor's office?" Her postscript to this story was: "It is humiliating when you get put through that. You don't want to go see a doctor after that."

Women in this study were clear in saying that their experiences of prejudicial behaviors limited the field of health care options available to them:

- I can't get the same quality of care as somebody who is white. I can't get the same quality of care as somebody who is straight. Compound that with the fact that I don't have money. I don't have insurance. What if I fall ill? It is a frightening thing. It is almost the kind of fear I can't even talk about.

Negative experiences with providers drove many of them away, exiled them from health care:

- Obviously, if you don't have the money, if you don't have health insurance, you don't have access to health care. But lesbians have other layers to the problem of access. If you go in for health care and you get abused because of who you are, you are not going to go. If you have been mistreated because you are lesbian, because you are female, because you are poor, because you are a woman of color, you are going to wait, and you are going to wait, and you are going to wait. And you are going to avoid going in until the very last minute.

Actions to Reduce Prejudice

Participants were adamant about changes that must occur to assure lesbians of color their safety and self-respect in health care encounters:

- As women, as lesbians, as people of color, we have these rotten health care experiences. And we get through them. Somehow, by our creativity and our ability to heal, we get through them. Sometimes we even make sure that the same thing doesn't happen to us twice. But what I believe is that there is no real progress until we know this will never happen to another woman again. It is not enough for me to be so clever that I don't get caught in a trap when I go in for health care. I want there to be no traps there, so nobody has to get caught.

This woman expresses a particular understanding of the danger and humiliation experienced by lesbians of color in health care encounters. She sees "traps" that cause deeply personal, privatized wounds. But these "traps" do not simply affect individuals; they have broader consequences. The "rotten health care experiences" she refers to represent structural patterns of health care delivery reinforcing marginalized women's perceptions that when they seek care, they do so as "other," as outsiders.

Another participant argued the insufficiency of piecemeal efforts to help individual providers become more "sensitive," and called for actions at the structural level to stop the prejudice:

- The whole system is inaccessible to me and people like me because of the homophobia, and the racism, and the sexism, to say nothing of inability to pay. Lesbians have worked hard to try to make inroads into mainstream health care, to get nurses and doctors over their shock and dismay. But a totally new system of health care is the bottom line. It just doesn't work to go decade after decade after decade putting all our efforts into trying to get a little bit of sensitivity from individual providers. Systems have to change. The system of education for nurses and doctors and the system of health care delivery have to stop imbuing, tolerating, and reinforcing prejudice.

Lesbians of color in this study were critical of the status quo, yet hopeful that things could be different. One woman summed it up this way:

- What the health care field really needs are more humanitarian advances, not technological advances. Providers who are more human, more sensitive. Health care is God's work. When health care providers are helping people who are sick and ailing, their hearts need to be there. The work is taking care of beings that are very God-like, no matter if we are poor, if we are lesbian, if we are Black, if we are fat or skinny. Rather than begrudge us, providers need to see their skills as a gift. They are very blessed to have the hands and the intelligence and the heart to do the work.

Another advised:

- Health care providers need to welcome lesbians of color in a way that makes us feel like family. What is imperative to stem the tide of prejudice that women of color suffer is for nurses and doctors to decide: We are going to take care of you like a sister would take care of a sister.

CONCLUSION

According to results of this qualitative study, lesbians of color contend with many interactional stimuli in health care. In the midst of any single encounter with a health care provider, they might have to decipher heterosexist remarks, steel themselves against racist epithets, counter undermining remarks insinuating gender inferiority, and heal from blows to their self-esteem as they are badgered about their deservedness as uninsured clients. One woman explained, "I feel that the negative attitudes I have encountered in health care have to do with every part of who I am; being lesbian, being a woman, being poor, being brown, being fat, being asthmatic." As lesbians of color tell it, vigilance and self-protection in all these areas are essential for their safety in health care encounters (Stevens, 1994b).

Within systems of health services as they are today, providers may spend years caring for impoverished women of color and not gain significant insight about the experiential perspectives of these clients. Providers may consider themselves familiar with the lifeways of persons who are actually simply behaving according to providers' expectations in order to get the service they need with a minimum of friction. And they will not see the clients who have been so traumatized in health care encounters that they change providers, or simply stop seeking help altogether. Without creating opportunities for real dialogue and the exchange of storied information, providers will continue to have blind spots that keep them from knowing how clients are really perceiving them and the services they are trying to deliver. Furthermore, until providers take action to stop themselves and their colleagues from behaving in harmful, frightening, and disrespectful ways, lesbians of color and other persons marginalized from the societal center cannot possibly risk changing their cautionary stance toward health care (Ferguson, Gever, Minh-ha, & West, 1990).

Storytelling humanizes research and practice. Basing our science of women's health on women's storied experiences holds great potential for the empowerment of women and the enhancement of health care services. Through women's narratives, we can learn concretely what their struggles are, what resources they need, and how health care providers' behaviors need to change. Study participants gave testimony to the effects of prejudice in face-to-face health care interactions. Evidence from their stories strongly suggests that if we wish to improve access to health services, those in the health care field must address race, class, gender, and sexual orientation prejudice in health care interactions, acknowledging the role discriminatory behavior plays in diminishing the availability of health care, not only to lesbians, but to the many other populations who do not fit normative stereotypes. Health care providers have lost credibility as witnesses and protectors of clients and we need to get it back. It is a sacred trust.

I conclude with one participant's message to health care providers:

- Don't make assumptions about me or anybody else. Take your chalkboard and wipe it clean every time you enter into conversation with a new patient. Go in with clear eyes and pure heart, understanding that we are all persons, even though the way we are in the world is different. When we are cut, we all bleed. Demonstrate to us that you are keeping that internal chalkboard clean by being conscious of how you talk with us, how you behave. You might say you don't have time. I say time is relative. There is always time to treat other people like human beings.

REFERENCES

Biernacki, P., & Waldorf, D. (1981). Snowball sampling: Problems and techniques of chain referral sampling. *Sociological Methods Research, 10*(2), 141-163.

Briggs, C. L. (1986). *Learning how to ask: A socio-linguistic appraisal of the role of the interview in social science research.* New York: Cambridge University Press.

Ferguson, R., Gever, M., Minh-ha, T., & West, C. (Eds.). (1990). *Out there: Marginalization and contemporary cultures.* Cambridge, MA: MIT Press.

Hall, J. M., & Stevens, P. E. (1991). Rigor in feminist research. *Advances in Nursing Science, 13*(3), 16-29.

Hall, J. M., Stevens, P. E., & Meleis, A. I. (1994). Marginalization: A guiding concept for valuing diversity in nursing knowledge development. *Advances in Nursing Science, 16*(4), 23-41.

hooks, b. (1984). *Feminist theory: From margin to center.* Boston, MA: South End Press.

Labov, W., & Waletzky, J. (1967). Narrative analysis: Oral versions of personal experience. In J. Helm (Ed.), *Essays on the verbal and visual arts: Proceedings of the 1966 annual spring meeting of the American Ethnological Society* (pp. 12-44). Seattle, WA: University of Washington Press.

Liaschenko, J. (1993). Feminist ethics and cultural ethos: Revisiting a nursing debate. *Advances in Nursing Science, 15*(4), 71-81.

Mishler, E. G. (1986). *Research interviewing: Context and narrative.* Cambridge, MA: Harvard University Press.

Polanyi, L. (1985). *Telling the American story: A structural and cultural analysis of conversational storytelling.* Norwood, NJ: Ablex.

Richardson, L. (1988). The collective story: Postmodernism and the writing of sociology. *Sociological Focus, 21*(3), 199-208.

Riessman, C. K. (1987). When gender is not enough: Women interviewing women. *Gender and Society, 1*(2), 172-207.

Riessman, C. K. (1993). *Narrative analysis: Qualitative research methods* (Vol. 30). Newbury Park, CA: Sage.

Stevens, P. E. (1993). Marginalized women's access to health care: A feminist narrative analysis. *Advances in Nursing Science, 16*(2), 39-56.

Stevens, P. E. (1994a). Lesbians' health-related experiences of care and noncare. *Western Journal of Nursing Research, 16*(6), 639-659.

Stevens, P. E. (1994b). Protective strategies of lesbian clients in health care environments. *Research in Nursing and Health, 17*(3), 217-229.

Stevens, P. E. (1996). Lesbians and doctors: Experiences of solidarity and domination in health care settings. *Gender & Society, 10*(1), 24-41.

U.S. Department of Labor. (1991). *Average annual pay levels in metropolitan areas, 1990.* Washington, DC: Bureau of Labor Statistics.

Room for Improvement: Communication Between Lesbians and Primary Care Providers

Jocelyn C. White
Valerie T. Dull

SUMMARY. In small studies lesbians report avoiding health care because of difficulty communicating with providers. This study examines lesbians' perceptions of communication with medical and alternative primary care providers using a statewide self-administered survey of members of a lesbian community organization. Univariate and bivariate statistics were used to analyze lesbians' perceptions of communication with their primary care provider about sexual orientation, difficult issues, and health issues important to les-

---

Jocelyn C. White, MD, FACP, FAAPP, is Assistant Professor of medicine at the Oregon Health Sciences University and faculty of the General Internal Medicine Training Program at Legacy Good Samaritan Hospital. Valerie T. Dull, PhD, is a member of the adjunct faculty at Portland State University and in the School of Professional Psychology at Pacific University. She currently is sole owner of Headway Consulting in Portland, Oregon. In the past she has been a senior analyst at the Institute for Social Science Research at UCLA and has been involved in health-care policy research for several national organizations.

Address correspondence to: Jocelyn C. White, Department of Medicine, Legacy Good Samaritan Hospital, 1015 NW 22nd Avenue, R-200, Portland, OR 97210-3079.

This project was funded by the Lesbian Health Fund, a project of the Gay and Lesbian Medical Association.

[Haworth co-indexing entry note]: "Room for Improvement: Communication Between Lesbians and Primary Care Providers." White, Jocelyn C., and Valerie T. Dull. Co-published simultaneously in *Journal of Lesbian Studies* (The Haworth Press, Inc.) Vol. 2, No. 1, 1998, pp. 95-110; and: *Gateways to Improving Lesbian Health and Health Care: Opening Doors* (ed: Christy M. Ponticelli) The Haworth Press, Inc., 1998, pp. 95-110; and: *Gateways to Improving Lesbian Health and Health Care: Opening Doors* (ed: Christy M. Ponticelli) Harrington Park Press, an imprint of The Haworth Press, Inc., 1998, pp. 95-110. Single or multiple copies of this article are available for a fee from The Haworth Document Delivery Service [1-800-342-9678, 9:00 a.m. - 5:00 p.m. (EST). E-mail address: getinfo@haworth.com].

bians. Of 324 respondents, 31% received primary care from alternative providers and 90% are "out" to one or more providers. Respondents who were "out" to their primary care provider were more likely to seek health and preventive care ($p \leq .05$), more likely to have ever had a Pap smear ($p \leq .02$), and more likely to be comfortable discussing sensitive issues ($p \leq .0001$). Respondents rated alternative providers easier to communicate with than M.D.s (4.53 vs. 3.99, $p \leq .001$). They reported being more open about sexual orientation (4.58 vs. 4.05, $p \leq .001$) and more comfortable discussing difficult issues (4.08 vs. 3.61, $p \leq .001$) with alternative providers. Respondents believe alternative providers understand lesbian health needs better than medical doctors (4.21 vs. 3.45, $p \leq .001$). Lesbians appear to be motivated to disclose sexual orientation to their primary care providers and disclosure is associated with positive health behaviors. Medical doctors appear to need improvement in their skills in communicating with lesbians so that important medical and psychosocial information can be shared. *[Article copies available for a fee from The Haworth Document Delivery Service: 1-800-342-9678. E-mail address: getinfo@haworth.com]*

Talk with lesbian patients as the courageous women they are. Every one has a story, a struggle and special stressors.

–Survey Respondent

INTRODUCTION

Lesbians may engage in certain health risk behaviors more than their heterosexual counterparts (Bradford, Ryan & Rothblum, 1994; Bybee, 1990; Kovar & Poe, 1985; McKirnan & Peterson, 1989; National Health Survey, 1987; National Survey on Drug Abuse, 1992; Robertson & Schacter, 1981; Skinner & Otis, 1992). These behaviors include smoking, heavy use of alcohol, unsafe sex, and avoidance of breast cancer screening and Pap tests. In addition, lesbians may have a higher body mass index than their heterosexual counterparts (Bradford et al., 1994; National Health and Nutrition Examination Survey, 1976-80). Therefore, lesbians may be at increased risk for breast, lung, cervical, head and neck, and colon cancers, as well as cardiovascular disease and HIV infection. Studies have also suggested that lesbians may be at increased risk of depression, suicidal ideation (Gillow & Davis, 1987; Goodwin, 1973) and alcohol abuse (Bloomfield, 1993; Lewis, Saghir & Robins, 1982). Lesbian patients may need specifically tailored counselling on such difficult or sensitive issues as sexual orientation confusion (Anstett, Kierman & Brown, 1987; Schneider, 1989), domestic violence (Renzetti, 1988; Schilit, Lie & Montagne, 1990; Schilit, Lie, Montagne & Reyes, 1991) sexual assault and abuse (Duncan, 1990), hate crimes (Gross, Aurand & Addessa, 1988; D'Augelli, 1989; Herek, 1989; National Gay and Lesbian Task Force, 1986), and depression (Cochran & Mays, 1994; Feinleib, 1989).

Unfortunately, many lesbians report that their doctors are not sensitive to or knowledgeable about these health risks and counselling needs (Smith, Johnson & Guenther, 1985). Some lesbians seek health care but are uncomfortable with the provider patient relationship and therefore do not disclose important information (Trippet & Bain, 1992). Others report avoiding health care and screening altogether when providers are not sensitive to their needs. Sixty-seven percent or more of lesbians surveyed report they are unable to disclose their sexual orientation ("come out") to their physician (Bybee, 1990; Cochran & Mays, 1988). Forty percent of those surveyed believe their care would be negatively affected by disclosing their sexual orientation (Johnson, Guenther, Laube & Keettel, 1981). Twenty to seventy-five percent of lesbians report negative responses from a health care provider after disclosure of sexual orientation (Stevens & Hall, 1988; Warshafsky, 1992). Likewise, forty percent of physicians in one study were sometimes or often uncomfortable providing care to lesbian and gay patients (Mathews, Booth, Turner & Kessler, 1986).

Based on these limited reports, lesbians may avoid health care, especially preventive care as a result of reluctance to disclose their sexual orientation or difficulty in communicating with their primary care provider. They also may fail to obtain important screening and risk factor counselling from their provider, either because of past or feared future difficulties. We have designed this large sample, state-wide survey to investigate lesbians' current communication with their primary care providers. One purpose of this study was to develop a greater understanding of lesbians' disclosure of sexual orientation to their primary care providers, their comfort in communicating and any relationship of sexual orientation disclosure to health behaviors. A second purpose was to discover whether communication plays a role in lesbians' reported preference for alternative providers (Trippet & Bain, 1992; Warshafsky, 1992).

METHODS

Sample

Respondents to the survey were from a convenience sample of two sources, a conference and a mailing list. The first source was a gathering of 70 people at a lesbian health care conference sponsored by the Lesbian Community Project in autumn 1994. The organization is a community-based social and political group based in Portland, Oregon, with lesbian members throughout the state. Participants at the conference were asked by a speaker and organization leaders to complete a questionnaire about lesbian health and return it to a drop box located at the registration desk. As the participants were likely to be on the mailing list, they were asked not to complete a second survey if they were to receive one in the mail. The second source was the readership of the Lesbian Community Project newsletter distributed to 1,000 addresses throughout the state of Oregon. Questionnaires were added by a mailing house to the monthly mailing of the newsletter in autumn, 1994. Investigators did not have access to the confidential mailing list. The instructions asked readers to complete and return the questionnaire in the self-addressed stamped envelope which was provided. Nonprobability samples of this type are often necessary with special populations when a sample frame is difficult or impossible to generate (Babbie, 1990).

Questionnaires

The questionnaire instrument consisted of a four page series of items divided into four sections. The first section pertained to health issues: breast, cervical, colon, ovarian, and lung cancer, smoking, alcohol use, drug use, weight, nutrition, exercise, coming out, hate crimes, domestic violence, sexual abuse, discrimination, parenting, stress management, menopause, depression, suicide, heart disease, HIV/AIDS, chronic fatigue syndrome, and high blood pressure. Respondents were asked to rate the importance of these issues to lesbians and to rate associated comfort levels when discussing each of these topics with primary care providers. Additional questions in this first section asked about alcohol consumption, health screening tests and smoking behaviors. The second section asked questions about the ease or difficulty of obtaining health care and general patterns of health seeking behaviors. Respondents were asked questions about their ease and comfort in communication with primary care providers and how open about their sexual orientation they were with these providers. This section also asked the respondent to identify her primary care provider as either a medical doctor, naturopathic doctor, chiropractic doctor, nurse practitioner, or "other." The third section asked about degrees of comfort in discussions of difficult issues and aspects about a provider they would consider important if they had to discuss sensitive issues. The last section asked questions about general demographic information and for any open-ended comments.

Analyses

When all questionnaires had been returned, numeric and text information were entered into a computer readable format and subjected to statistical analysis using SPSS for Windows, Release 6.0. The first step in the analysis was to tabulate univariate statistics describing the distributions for individual items. Items were separately tabulated for conference and mail-in samples to look for significant differences in these groups. Subsequently, bivariate analyses were used to compare groups of women who use M.D.s as primary care providers and those who use other health professionals.

RESULTS

Response rates were 71% (n = 50) for the conference group and 27% (n = 274) for the mail-in group from the newsletter. While the response rate for the mail-in group is undesirably low, it is not unusual for a one-time anonymous mailing (Fowler, 1988). One questionnaire was not received in time for data entry and was thus excluded from analysis. Partially complete questionnaires were included in the data set with missing values substituted for nonresponse to particular items.

The conference and mail-in data were analyzed for significant differences on both continuous and categorical responses. Conference respondents were significantly different in individual unpaired t-tests, rating almost every issue in the list of health issues as "more important" (with the exception of "coming out" and "depression," which were not different because they were highly rated by both groups). Moreover, there were significantly more minority women in the conference group (30% vs. 10% minority/other, chi-square = 46.9, $p \leq .0001$) and significantly fewer women covered by health insurance in the conference group (20% vs. 6% no coverage, chi-square = 17.1, $p \leq .05$) (Table 1). Of note, the Oregon Health Plan (federal Medicaid waiver) was in effect during this study and purports to ensure that over 90% of the Oregon population has health care coverage.

However, respondents were not significantly different on any of the other issues being targeted for investigation in this study, including comfort with communication, health screening and risks, and type of provider. Therefore, while it would appear that conference attenders were more highly polarized in their ratings with respect to commitment on important issues and differed somewhat on demographics, the data were combined for further analysis. The organization could not provide characteristics of the mailing list.

TABLE 1

SAMPLE DIFFERENCES			
	Conference (N = 70)	Mailing (N = 1000)	
Response Rate	71%	27%	
Minority Women	30%	10%	($p \leq .0001$)
No Insurance	20%	6%	($p \leq .05$)

Univariate results describing the respondent sample are shown in Table 2. The mean age for these women was 41.0 years ($SD = 8.5$) and 84.6% (n = 274) were Caucasian. The level of education for most respondents was exceptionally high. The majority (58.6%) reported having more than a college-level education. Most women were working full time (70.1%) and carried health insurance of some type (89.5%).

Most respondents (65.3%) reported that they had primary care providers who were medical doctors, but, surprisingly, 31.6% of respondents used alternative providers such as naturopaths (13%), chiropractors (3%), nurse practitioners (8%), or others (7%). Respondents reported having primary care providers who were physician assistants, herbalists, acupuncturists, massage therapists, psychic healers, and one clairvoyant. Three percent had no primary care provider.

A large number of respondents are "out" to one or more of their health care providers (90%). Fifty percent are out to all providers, 29% to some and 12% to their primary care provider only. Three percent said, "I think they know"; 4% said, "I don't know if they know"; and 3% are out to none. Of the 90% of women out, most of them (92%) raised the issue themselves with the provider. Of the women with medical doctors, 68% opened the topic themselves and 4% of their doctors did. Of those with alternative providers, 62% opened the topic and 8% of their providers did. Seven and 20% of respondents with medical and alternative providers respectively reported other ways in which sexual orientation was disclosed. Many respondents reported "coming out" during the visit when the provider asked, "What kind of birth control do you use?" Other ways that respondents said the provider learned of their sexual orientation included, "It was on my medical history form"; "He already knew because he treated my partner"; "My place of employment is a dead-giveaway"; and "It's a lesbian clinic and I'm extremely blatant so it may not

TABLE 2

SAMPLE CHARACTERISTICS			
Age	range	18-71	
	average	41	
	standard deviation	8.5	
Gender	female	322	99.4%
	male	0	0
	other ("butch")	1	0.3
Relationships	single	96	29.6%
	living with partner	167	51.5
	living apart	46	14.2
	separated	7	2.2
	widowed	1	0.3
Legal Marital Status	single	243	75%
	married	5	1.5
	divorced	62	19.1
	separated	1	0.3
Sexual Partners	only women	77	23.8%
	mostly women	149	46.0
	men and women equally	29	9.0
	mostly men	43	13.3
	only men	2	0.6
	none	1	0.3
	other	12	3.7
Sexual Orientation Identity	lesbian	287	88.6%
	bisexual	15	4.6
	no identity	6	1.9
	other	4	1.2
	missing	12	3.7

TABLE 2 (continued)

Ethnicity/Race	Caucasian	274	84.6%
	African American	12	3.7
	Asian/Pacific Islander	5	1.5
	Latino/Hispanic	2	0.6
	Native American	2	0.6
	multi-racial	7	2.2
	other	13	4.0
Schooling	less than high school	2	0.6%
	high school	4	1.2
	some college	58	17.9
	four years college	59	18.2
	more than college	190	58.6
Work	full time	227	70.1%
	part time	28	8.6
	looking for work	12	3.7
	student	9	2.8
	home/child care	2	0.6
	retired	5	1.6
	disabled	5	1.5
	other	15	4.6
Health Insurance	yes	290	89.5%
	no	28	8.6
	don't know	1	0.3
	other	1	0.3

have actually been discussed, just like straights don't discuss being straight with their straight doctor."

Interestingly, 74.0% (233) of respondents found it easy or extremely easy to communicate with their primary care provider, and 26.0% (82) found it only moderately or not easy to communicate with their primary care provider. When asked whether their primary care provider understood lesbians' health needs, 59.4% (170) believed providers understood them well or very well, 20.6% (59) moderately well, and 19.9 (57) not well or not at all.

We looked at several of these primary care health issues in relation to whether the patient was out to the primary care provider. Respondents who were out to their primary care provider were more likely to seek health and preventive care (chi-square (5) = 13.27, $p \leq .02$), have ever had a Pap test (chi-square (1) = 7.38, $p \leq .007$) and currently be a non-smoker (chi-square (1) = 10.02, $p \leq .002$). They were also more likely to report a comfortable sexual orientation disclosure discussion (chi-square (6) = 130.58, $p < .0001$), general ease of communication with their provider (chi-square (4) = 64.79, $p < .0001$), having a primary care provider who understands lesbian health needs (chi-square (4) = 94.21, $p < .0001$), and feeling comfortable discussing difficult issues with their primary care provider (chi-square (4) = 41.06, $p < .0001$).

As shown in Figure 1, in general respondents rated alternative providers easier to communicate with than medical doctors. Respondents felt they could be more open about their sexual orientation and more comfortable in discussing difficult issues with alternative providers. Respondents believed that alternative providers understood lesbian health needs better. They did, however, find no difference in the comfort of the actual coming out discussion comparing medical doctors and alternative providers.

We asked respondents how comfortable they were the last time they discussed a difficult issue with their primary care provider: 56.2% (177) were comfortable or extremely comfortable, 21.0% (66) were moderately comfortable, 12.1% (38) were uncomfortable, 10.8% (34) responded in another manner. Most of those responding "other" said they hadn't had a difficult discussion with their provider.

For those respondents who were uncomfortable in discussing a difficult issue, 27.9% believed it was because of something about themselves that caused the difficulty, and 30.4% believed something about the doctor caused the difficulty, although some respondents wrote about feeling rushed or uncomfortable about the issue, many comments related to sexual orientation. Speaking of the provider, some respondents wrote, "They had discomfort about women's issues"; "She assumed I was heterosexual"; "She was not used to people coming out to her"; "She is not a lesbian and doesn't really understand even though she is not judgmental"; "I asked about lesbian safer sex. She didn't know what to tell me except to call [the local AIDS community resource]"; and "I had an abdominal lump. My mother died of cancer. My primary barely touched it. I think it's because she thinks I'm a lesbian." Speaking of themselves, some lesbians wrote, "I was worried a little about judgements"; "I found it embarrassing"; "I

FIGURE 1. Communication with the Primary Care Provider

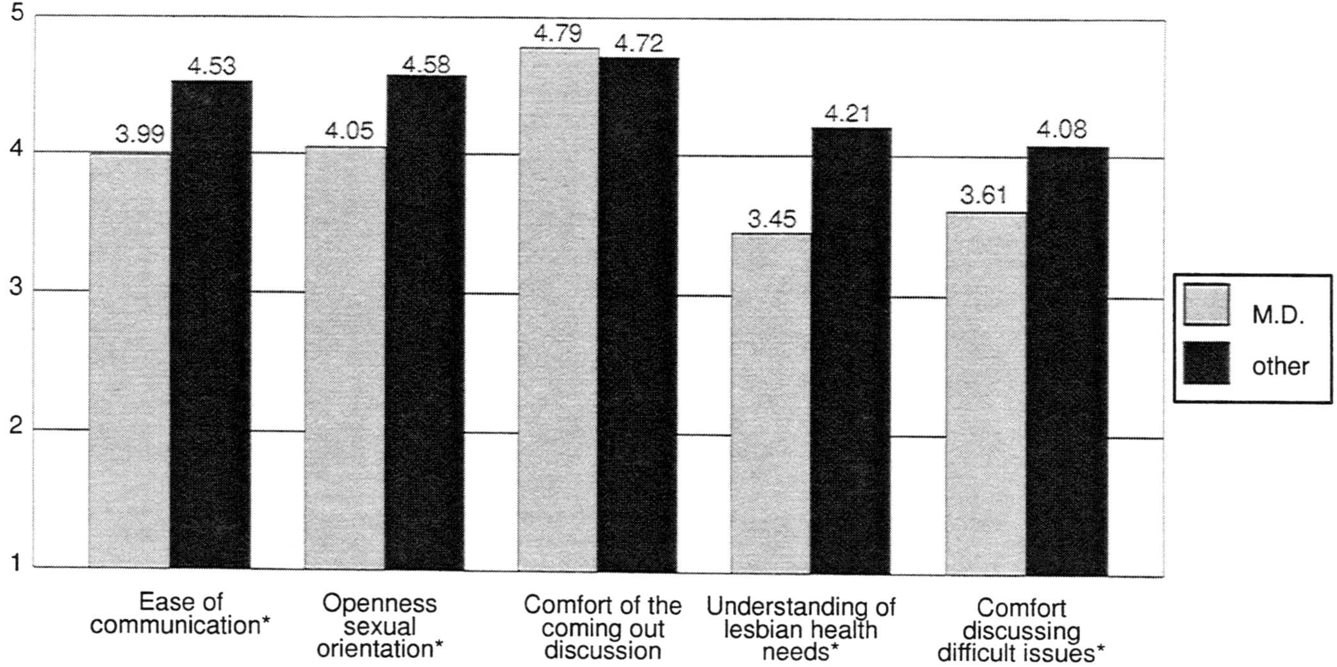

Average Likert Ratings by Provider (1 = not at all; 5 = very easy/well)
*** indicates differences are significant ($p \leq .001$)**
t-test for Equality of Means, 2-tailed significance

was hesitant to come out temporarily"; "The difficulty is probably mine because of preconceived ideas about homophobia"; "I find it difficult to talk about health issues, especially if I'm scared"; and, "Until I tell her I'm a lesbian, I can't expect good care–completely."

Respondents were asked to rate the importance of certain provider characteristics when deciding to discuss difficult issues with that provider (Likert scale with 1 = "not at all" and 5 = "extremely important"). Respondents rated communication style as most important and provider gender as second most important: communication style (4.56); gender (4.30); sexual orientation (2.74); age (2.57); other (2.27) (philosophy most often cited); religion (1.88); race (1.81); weight (1.65); and physical abilities (1.62). Of note, sexual orientation was not among the highly-rated characteristics.

The top ten health issues important to lesbians from a list of 25 such issues, as ranked by respondents, include biological and psychosocial topics (Figure 2). Respondents rated alternative providers significantly higher on comfort in discussing discrimination, hate crimes, coming out, alcohol use and drug use compared to medical doctors.

DISCUSSION

In contrast to previous work, lesbians in this study appear to be highly motivated to disclose sexual orientation to their primary care providers. The vast majority of lesbians in this study had done so. Still, over a quarter of respondents had difficulty communicating with their primary care providers about difficult or sensitive issues. Often the difficulty arose because of sexual orientation issues. This is a significant finding considering respondents rated communication style the most important provider characteristic. In addition, a large portion believe that their primary care provider lacks knowledge of lesbian health issues. These figures are of concern because current medical teaching recognizes that primary care providers need the skills to communicate sensitively and the knowledge to provide competent care for lesbian patients (White & Levinson, 1995).

Interestingly, the rate of sexual orientation disclosure in this study is considerably higher than that previously reported (Bradford et al., 1994; Bybee, 1990; Dardick & Grady, 1980). Perhaps these respondents were more motivated to disclose because of the education they had received through their community newsletter. Perhaps they were influenced by the increasing visibility of lesbian and gay issues in the news media. Perhaps the change in the social climate in the decade since previous studies has encouraged higher rates of disclosure. If the community newsletter played a role in this disclosure, there are implications for community-based health

FIGURE 2. Ten Most Important Health Issues to Lesbians and Comfort Discussing Them with the Primary Care Provider

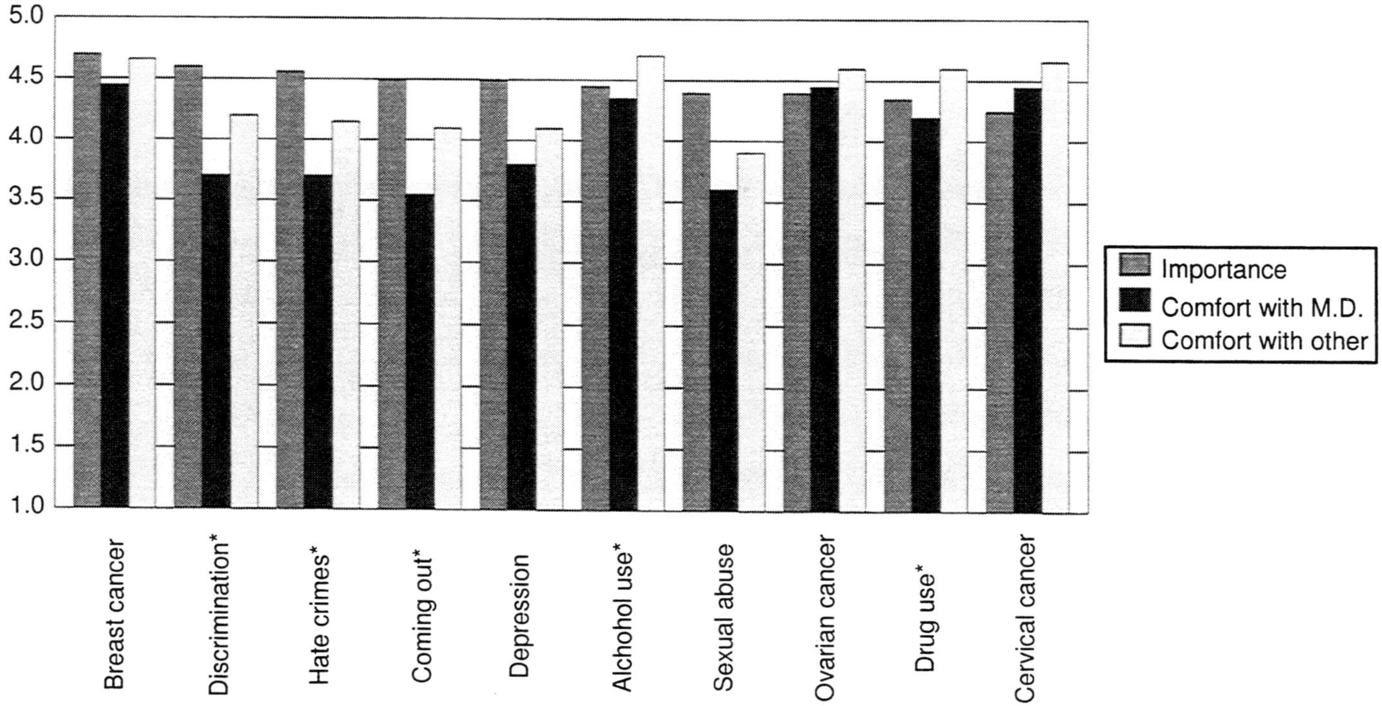

Average Likert Ratings (1 = not at all; 5 = extremely important/comfortable)
*** indicates comfort values significantly different ($p \leq .02$)**
t-test for Equality of Means, 2-tailed significance

education of lesbians. Such education may encourage sexual orientation disclosure and increase the amount of information exchanged between lesbians and their primary care providers. Because sampling was challenging for this group, these questions cannot be definitively answered by this study.

We found that lesbians disclosed sexual orientation equally to medical providers and alternative providers but were able to be more open with the alternative providers and found they had a generally easier communication style. In addition, study respondents believed alternative providers had a better knowledge of lesbian health issues. We do not know how many lesbian providers there were in each group. But if there were more lesbian providers in the alternative group, this may have affected the results. The good communication ratings which alternative providers received may have created an illusion of a greater knowledge base among alternative providers in the minds of respondents. We have considered that the presence of colleges of naturopathic, chiropractic and Oriental medicine in Oregon and the apparent large numbers of alternative providers in this state may have affected our results in ways that would not be found in other regions. Their greater presence does, however, provide a larger population of respondents who have had exposure to and can make judgement about alternative providers.

The importance of sexual orientation disclosure to the health of a lesbian is supported by our findings. Those respondents who were out to their primary care providers were more likely to seek early and preventive care, more likely to have had Pap smears, and were more comfortable in discussing difficult issues. While no causation can be inferred from these results, they appear to indicate that there is an association between being able to discuss sexual orientation successfully with the primary care provider and improved health-seeking, screening, and sharing of sensitive health information.

This study has several limitations. First, it is not comprised of a random sample of lesbians from the community. The task of recruiting vulnerable or "hidden" populations poses unique challenges for the investigator. Convenience samples are sometimes required. Two advantages of this study are the broad community base and the large numbers of respondents to the survey. Very few community-based surveys have involved these numbers of lesbian respondents. In fact, most of the research studies exploring lesbians' communication with their primary care providers have involved small, snowball samples used for univariate and qualitative analysis. The ideal survey would include women of all sexual orientations for comparison purposes. We encourage survey researchers to include sexual orientation items in survey instruments for all large-scale health surveys.

Second, this sample may not be typical of lesbians in the greater population in that these women were members of a community organization who have for several years been reading a newsletter about lesbian health issues, the importance of regular screening, and good primary care. If the newsletter has influenced responses, the problems highlighted in this study may be even more important for the general population of lesbians. This study provides us with updated information on what has been in general a strained relationship between lesbians and their primary care providers. Compared to previous studies, lesbians have increased their willingness to disclose sexual orientation to providers. If this observed change is a result of an evolving social climate, we may expect to see it reflected in other recent surveys. If this increase in willingness to disclose is due to targeted health education by the community organization, an argument can be made that similar education would benefit lesbians elsewhere.

Although this study points out several apparent improvements in the relationship between lesbians and their primary care providers, clearly there is still room for more improvement on the part of providers, especially medical doctors. This study suggests that sensitive communication between providers and patients that does not assume heterosexuality has a positive impact on lesbians' willingness to disclose sexual orientation information, and disclosure of sexual orientation is associated with seeking health care early, getting Pap smears, and discussing other sensitive issues. Providers now have specific health-related incentives to ask questions and phrase intake forms in a way that does not assume heterosexual orientation and demonstrates knowledge of lesbian health issues. Such knowledge is now widely available (Denenberg, 1995; O'Hanlan, 1995; Rankow, 1995; White & Levinson, 1993; White & Levinson, 1995). Only through improved use of specific communication skills (White & Levinson, 1995) and possession of an adequate knowledge base can providers care for lesbian patients in a sensitive, competent manner.

REFERENCES

Anstett, Richard; Kierman, Martin; & Brown, Richard. (1987). The gay-lesbian patient and the family physician. *Journal of Family Practice, 25*(4), 339-44.

Babbie, Earl. (1990). *Survey research methods* (2nd Ed.). Belmont, California: Wadsworth Publishing.

Bloomfield, Kim. (1993). A comparison of alcohol consumption between lesbians and heterosexual women in an urban population. *Drug and Alcohol Dependence, 33*, 257-69.

Bradford, Judith; Ryan, Caitlin & Rothblum, Esther. (1994). National Lesbian Health Care Survey: Implications for mental health care. *Journal of Consulting and Clinical Psychology 62*, 228-42.

Bybee, D. (March, 1990). Michigan Lesbian Health Survey: A report to the Michigan Organization for Human Rights and the Michigan Department of Public Health. Michigan Department of Health & Human Services.

Cochran, Susan & Mays Vickie. (1994). Depressive distress among homosexually active African American men and women. *American Journal of Psychiatry, 151*(4), 524-29.

Cochran, Susan & Mays, Vickie. (1988). Disclosure of sexual preference to physicians by black lesbian and bisexual women. *Western Journal of Medicine, 149*(5), 616-619.

Dardick, Larry & Grady, Kathleen. (1980). Openness between gay persons and health professionals. *Annals of Internal Medicine, 93*(1), 115-119.

D'Augelli, Anthony. (1989). Lesbians' and gay men's experience of discrimination and harassment in a university community. *American Journal of Community Psychology, 17*(3), 317-21.

Denenberg, Risa. (1995). Report on Lesbian Health. *Women's Health Issues, 5*(2), 1-11.

Duncan, David. (1990). Prevalence of sexual assault victimization among heterosexual and gay/lesbian university students. *Psychological Reports, 66*, 65-6.

Feinleib, Marcia. (1989). Report of the Secretary's Task Force on Youth Suicide. Rockville, Maryland: U.S. Department of Health and Human Services.

Fowler, Floyd. (1988). Survey research methods: Applied social research methods series. Volume 1. Newbury Park, California: Sage Publications.

Gillow, Kim & Davis, Linda. (1987). Lesbian stress and coping methods. *Journal of Psychosocial Nursing & Mental Health Services, 25*(9), 28-32.

Goodwin, Donald. (1973). Alcohol in suicide and homicide. *Quarterly Journal of Studies on Alcohol, 34*, 144-56.

Gross, Larry; Aurand, Steven & Addessa, Rita. (1988). *Violence and discrimination against lesbian and gay people in Philadelphia and the Commonwealth of Pennsylvania*. Philadelphia, PA: Philadelphia Lesbian and Gay Task Force.

Herek, Gregory. (1989). Hate crimes against lesbians and gay men: issues for research and policy. *American Psychologist, 44*(6), 948-55.

Johnson, Susan; Guenther, Susan; Laube, Douglas & Keettel, William. (1981). Factors influencing lesbian gynecologic care: A preliminary study. *American Journal of Obstetrics & Gynecology, 140*, 20-8.

Kovar, Mary & Poe, Gail. (1985). National Health Interview Survey. U.S. Department of Health & Human Services (PHS) 85-1320. National Center for Health Statistics, Washington, D.C.

Lewis, Collins; Saghir, Marcel & Robins, Eli. (1982). Drinking patterns in homosexual and heterosexual women. *Journal of Clinical Psychiatry, 43*(7), 277-9.

Mathews, William; Booth, Mary; Turner, John & Kessler, Lois. (1986). Physician's attitudes toward homosexuality–survey of a California County Medical Society. *Western Journal of Medicine, 144*, 106-10.

McKirnan, David & Peterson, Peggy. (1989). Alcohol and drug use among homosexual men and women: Epidemiology and population characteristics. *Addictive Behaviors, 14*, 545-553.

National Gay and Lesbian Task Force. (1986). Kevin Berrill, Director, Violence Project. Anti-gay violence: causes, consequences, responses. Washington, D.C.

National Health Interview Survey. (1987).

National Health and Nutrition Examination Survey. (1976-80).

National Survey on Drug Abuse. (1992). U.S. Department of Health, Education & Welfare (ADM) 78-620. National Institute on Drug Abuse, Division of Research, Rockville, Maryland.

O'Hanlan, Katherine. (1995). Lesbian health and homophobia: Perspectives for the treating obstetrician/ gynecologist. *Current Problems in Obstetrics, Gynecology and Fertility, 18*(4), 94-133.

Rankow, Elizabeth. (1995). Lesbian Health Issues for the Primary Care Provider. *Journal of Family Practice, 40*(5), 486-493.

Renzetti, Claire. (1988). Violence in lesbian relationships: A preliminary analysis of causal factors. *Journal of Interpersonal Violence, 3*(4), 381-99.

Robertson, Patricia & Schacter, Julius. (1981). Failure to identify venereal disease in a lesbian population. *Sexually Transmitted Diseases, 8*(2), 75-6.

Schilit, Rebecca; Lie, Gwat-Yong; Montagne, Marilyn & Reyes, Lynn. (1991). Intergenerational transmission of violence in lesbian relationships. *Journal of Interpersonal Violence, 6*(1), 72-87.

Schilit, Rebecca; Lie, Gwat-Yong & Montagne, Marilyn. (1990). Substance use as a correlate of violence in intimate lesbian relationships. *Journal of Homosexuality, 19*(3), 51-65.

Schneider, Margaret. (1989). Sappho was a right-on adolescent: growing up lesbian. *Journal of Homosexuality, 17*(1-2), 111-30.

Skinner, William & Otis, Melanie. (July 1992). Trilogy Project: Research in the lesbian and gay community, 14th National Lesbian and Gay Health Conference, Los Angeles, California.

Smith, Elaine; Johnson, Susan & Guenther, Susan. (1985). Health care attitudes and experiences during gynecologic care among lesbians and bisexuals. *American Journal of Public Health, 75*(9), 1085-7.

Stevens, Patricia & Hall, Joanne. (1988). Stigma, health beliefs and experiences with health care in lesbian women. *Image: Journal of Nursing Scholarship, 20*(2), 69-73.

Trippet, Susan & Bain, Joyce. (1992). Reasons American lesbians fail to seek traditional health care. *Health Care for Women International, 13*, 145-53.

Warshafsky, Lynn. (April 1992). Lesbian health needs assessment: prepared for the Los Angeles Gay and Lesbian Community Service Center.

White, Jocelyn & Levinson, Wendy. (1995). Primary care of lesbian patients. In: Noble J. *Primary care and general medicine (2nd ed)*. St. Louis, MO: Mosby Year Book, 129A, (pp. 1696-1700.)

White, Jocelyn & Levinson, Wendy. (1993). Primary care of lesbian patients. *Journal of General Internal Medicine, 8*, 41-47.

Index

COSTS: Please figure your cost to order quality copies of an article.

1. Set-up charge per article: $8.00
   ($8.00 × number of separate articles) ________
2. Photocopying charge for each article:
   1-10 pages: $1.00 ________
   11-19 pages: $3.00 ________
   20-29 pages: $5.00 ________
   30+ pages: $2.00/10 pages ________
3. Flexicover (optional): $2.00/article ________
4. Postage & Handling: US: $1.00 for the first article/
   $.50 each additional article ________
   Federal Express: $25.00 ________
   Outside US: $2.00 for first article/
   $.50 each additional article ________
5. Same-day FAX service: $.35 per page ________

GRAND TOTAL: ____________

METHOD OF PAYMENT: (please check one)

❑ Check enclosed ❑ Please ship and bill. PO # ________________
(sorry we can ship and bill to bookstores only! All others must pre-pay)

❑ Charge to my credit card: ❑ Visa; ❑ MasterCard; ❑ Discover;
❑ American Express;

Account Number: ____________________ Expiration date: __________

Signature: ✗ ______________________________

Name: ____________________ Institution: ____________________

Address: ______________________________________

____

City: ____________________ State: ________ Zip: __________

Phone Number: ________________ FAX Number: ________________

MAIL or *FAX* THIS ENTIRE ORDER FORM TO:

Haworth Document Delivery Service
The Haworth Press, Inc.
10 Alice Street
Binghamton, NY 13904-1580

or FAX: 1-800-895-0582
or CALL: 1-800-342-9678
9am-5pm EST)